"Every healthcare provider who works with expectant families should be required to read this book. *Our Only Time* is a perfect blend of resources - heartbreaking stories from loss families, side by side with practical and essential information for those who care for them."

—KAYTEE FISHER, Registered Nurse and bereaved mother

"*Our Only Time* is a love letter to health professionals who work with parents whose babies have died. Written and edited by a mother who herself received quality bereavement care, this book doesn't tell caregivers what to do, but rather, provides insight and modeling largely in the form of powerful narratives written by bereaved parents who were deeply touched by the kind words, small gestures, and caring intentions of their caregivers. Each story imparts a lesson on what grieving parents find comforting, meaningful, and beneficial. For midwives, nurses, physicians, technicians, counselors, therapists, chaplains, and social workers, this heartfelt book offers clarity and inspiration for offering the care that parents crave; care that fosters their coping, adjustment, and transformational healing."

—DEBORAH L. DAVIS, PhD
Developmental Psychologist & Writer
Empty Cradle, Broken Heart: Surviving the Death of Your Baby
www.psychologytoday.com/blog/laugh-cry-live

"*Our Only Time* is a book of healing, hope and inspiration. As a nurse and a parent advocate, I am grateful for the powerful stories shared and the strategies offered for healthcare professionals. It truly is wonderful to be a part of a baby's birth. When death comes with birth there is a need for a greater compassion and empathy, a validation of the baby and an acknowledgment of the pain of the loss. *Our Only Time* is a wonderful appreciation to the caring professionals that serve families with a true presence and a reminder of the things needed to allow a family to care for and love their baby during such a short time."

—PATTI BUDNIK RN, BSN, CPLC Bereavement Care Manager
Share Pregnancy and Infant Loss Support

"*Our Only Time* is an exceptional resource for nurses as they guide parents through the unimaginable time of the loss of a child. As a labor and delivery nurse, it is difficult to know what to say or do to help. The personal stories on these pages share the heartache, but also the helpful actions that have made a difference in the darkest moments. Thank you, Amie, for your passion, for honoring the life of each of these little ones, and for showing us how to be a light in the darkness for our patients."

—WENDY RHOADS, Registered Nurse

"In writing *Our Only Time* Amie Lands has created an inspiring and heartfelt resource for both grieving parents and dedicated professionals who support these special families. This books serves two needs and meets both components with success; for parents to understand what professionals need to support them and for professionals to understand the path that grieving parents walk. Thank you, Amie, for sharing your personal journey and for reaching out to all those impacted by baby loss."

—CHERYL SALTER-ROBERTS,
Co-Founder, Grief Counselor and Educator
H.E.A.R.T.S. Baby Loss Support Program, Baby Steps Walk to Remember, BriarPatch Family Life Education Centre

"The strategies in this straightforward and heartfelt guide comes directly from parents who have survived the nightmare of losing a beloved child in pregnancy or soon after birth. These stories serve as a powerful reminder that every loss is different, as unique and individual as the people those children might have grown up to be."

—MARGOT FINN, *Ending a Wanted Pregnancy*

"*Our Only Time* is a powerful and important book that resonates with the voices of women for women and their families, voices spoken in requests to their health care providers. Amie Lands' work continues to contribute to our understanding of pregnancy and infant loss, and to assist caring others help us integrate our losses into our lives in meaningful ways."

—DEBORAH DAVIDSON, PhD, Associate Professor, editor and contributing author of *The Tattoo Project: Commemorative Tattoos, Visual Culture, and the Digital Archive*

"In Social Work practice, we strive to achieve the goals set out by the National Association of Social Workers' Code of Ethics. We often refer to social work as 'practice', not 'perfect'. Author, Amie Lands, offers Medical Social Workers the opportunity to deepen their practice through her heartfelt and practical book *Our Only Time*. It is impossible to fully prepare a practitioner to attend to the needs of families who have lost their baby because not only is the magnitude of pain they are feeling unfathomable to comprehend; moreover, each family will have their unique experience and process. As a Medical Social Worker, it is easy to feel completely overwhelmed and useless in a situation as heartbreaking, sensitive and consequently, of the utmost importance, as a family suffering under these circumstances. This is when the ego wants to do social work perfect and not practice. This seemingly insurmountable responsibility feels significantly more attainable thanks to the incredible series of stories Lands has compiled. Lands' book is simultaneously heartbreaking and uplifting as she chronicles stories of loss, surrender, love, and hope. We will never be perfect in this, but in reading this, we practice."

—CHLOE RUSCA DUNEGAN, Licensed Clinical Social Worker

ALSO BY AMIE LANDS

Navigating the Unknown: An Immediate Guide
When Experiencing the Loss of Your Baby

OUR ONLY
Time

STORIES OF PREGNANCY/INFANT LOSS
WITH STRATEGIES FOR HEALTH PROFESSIONALS

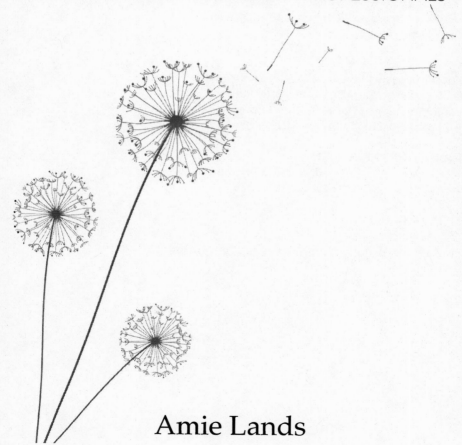

Amie Lands

Our Only Time is published by Kat Biggie Press.
www.katbiggiepress.com

Cover design by Michelle Fairbanks, Fresh Design
Book design by Alexa Bigwarfe, Write I Publish I Sell
Editing by Bridgett Harris, Triple B Writing Services
Author photograph by Seasyn McDowell

ISBN-13: 978-0-9994377-7-3
Library of Congress Control Number: 2017959842
First Edition: November 2017

10 9 8 7 6 5 4 3 2 1

For bulk orders, contact: amielandsauthor@gmail.com

In honor of every baby in this book,
I will forever wish you were here for your family to hold and watch grow.

Contents

Acknowledgements

WITH UTMOST GRATITUDE to the health professionals who hold the hands and hearts of families suffering this unimaginable loss, I sincerely thank you. Your ability to guide patients through such devastation with tender care will always be part of their story.

To the contributors of this book, your strength, your grace, and your love for your babies is breathtaking. Your willingness to share the most heartbreaking moment of your life in order to support other families is an incredible gift.

To the team that supported the creation of this book, thank you. Alexa Bigwarfe, Write, Publish, Sell; Bridgett Harris, Triple B Writing Services, LLC; Michelle Fairbanks, Fresh Design; and Seasyn McDowell, Seasyn McDowell Photography; I am so grateful for your professionalism, guidance, and support.

To my husband, Chris, and sons, Reid and Adam, I love you more than anything else in the whole wide world. I am so grateful for your unconditional love, gentle encouragement and neverending support. Thank you for the many hours that you allowed me to honor Ruthie Lou by writing this book.

And finally, a "thank you" will never be enough for the loving care that went far beyond patient at both Kaiser Health Foundation Oakland and George Mark Children's House. Your guidance, kindness, and respect you offered tremendously impacted the trajectory of my family's life, at a time when life as we knew it was ending. I honestly do not know that our hearts would have survived if it had not been for the grace you showed us. The memories that were created during our daughter's life are our most treasured moments. Thank you, for having the awareness to lovingly guide our family both during and after Ruthie Lou's life.

Foreword

AT ITS HEART, MEDICINE is a human endeavor; however, it is often challenging to care for patients within current medical systems while maintaining a sense of the personal. As a neonatologist, perinatal palliative care provider, bioethicist, and medical educator, I face the challenge every day. In medical education and training medical providers, we are challenged to impart the importance of looking beyond the pathophysiology to find the patient. The paradigm of medical education is that you learn about patients' disease processes by observing the pathology play out in "real life." Frequently, it is unrecognized that the patient teaches us about more than the disease.

Patient and family narratives are powerful teaching tools, and in her book, *Our Only Time*, Amie Lands provides us with an invaluable resource. In this collection of narratives and guidance for medical caregivers, she teaches us how to be better for our patients. Through their own words, we gain an extraordinary view into patients' lives and experiences. The honesty of these families and their willingness to share the most intimate, raw, painful, joyful, and sacred moments of their lives is humbling, and it is important that we honor them and hear them. As caregivers, our words matter and families often carry them for years. Names hold immense power and build a child's legacy. Our actions, or inactions, imprint in families' memories. Our tears, often shed in what we may regard as moments of weakness, are cherished by families who recognize them as the signs of love that they are. As medical providers, realizing the impact that we have on families can be an immense burden, and recognizing this, Amie Lands uses her experience and the knowledge and experience of others to provide us with guidance. *Our Only Time* is a gift for medical caregivers and their patients.

When I am teaching students, residents, and fellows, I often find myself telling stories about my patients and families. Sharing the experience of caring for a patient in order to emphasize important themes is natural in clinical education. In the tradition of medical apprenticeship, I am merely passing along what my patients have taught me. Families have taught me about patience, love and hope. Mothers have shown me what true strength and unconditional love look like. Fathers have demonstrated tenderness and fierce resolve to care for their families, and babies have taught me about resilience and finding joy and peace in the face of unimaginable pain. Each lesson makes me a better doctor for my next patient and family. *Our Only Time* provides readers with insight that could otherwise take years of clinical experience to encounter, and with this book, Amie Lands provides us with a narrative medicine "textbook," a meaningful experience of love, grief, and hope, and a useful practical guide to be better caregivers.

—CHRISTINE E BISHOP, MD, MA
Neonatologist, Medical Director of Neonatal/Perinatal Palliative Care
Wake Forest University School of Medicine, Brenner Children's Hospital

Preface

IN WRITING THIS BOOK, I have had many hesitations. I sheepishly wondered who I was to write this book when I have zero medical training. I do not work as a healthcare provider. I do not practice medicine. I do not have the years of education or the experience that you do, dear reader. So, why would anyone in the health profession listen to me?

As my ego interfered and put pause to the publishing of this book, I had to set my hesitation aside. For the last six years I have lived a life that I never imagined — nor would have chosen. I carried and birthed a child that lived only 33 days. I have the hard-earned education from experience that no other parent would want — one whose child has died. The life I lived ended the day that I was informed that my daughter would not survive off life support, when she was referred to as "incompatible with life". Those words changed the trajectory of my existence and created a new path. I had to learn how to enter the world again. My grief caused me to reconsider who I was and the impact I wanted to create in my lifetime.

Because of the loving-kindness of the professionals who cared for my family, I am now compelled to do the same to help bereaved parents in any way possible. I have a passion that I cannot deny. I may not have educational experience in the medical field, but I have valuable life experience. If I were a health professional wanting to learn how to best support my patients, I would want the words of those who have survived this loss to guide me. That is what you will find within these pages, words from parents who would rather not have this knowledge, but hope, through their stories, they will help another family experiencing loss.

I wrote this book, collected and compiled the stories included, so that you would know from the bottom of our broken hearts, how grateful families are to you for the gifts that you offer us in our deepest moments of despair. Whether a huge gesture or a kind word, every moment matters as life is falling apart. What you are observing is an entire lifetime in mere hours and if we are lucky, days that we have with our baby before we continue our life without them. We need you. We need your guidance, your expertise and mostly, we need your compassion.

"Health professionals", as written in this resource, encompasses any birth worker or professional including, but not limited to, surgeons, doctors, midwives, nurses, doulas, chaplains, social workers, child life specialists, counselors, therapists — any professional that handles mamas, babies, and grief following loss has been included. Together, this team collectively serves the needs of those while pregnant, during the time when families are able to hold their baby (if any time at all), and when re-entering life without their child.

I can only assume that when you entered this profession, you imagined supporting families through one of life's greatest moments, growing a family. However, as you have learned, there is an entire group of parents, bereaved parents, who do not receive a happy ending and whose lives devastatingly change the moment they learn that their child will or has died. Your ability to care for these patients with an open heart and empathy will drastically impact how they move forward in life.

This book is written in two parts. The first includes personal accounts from families. The second elaborates the lesson of their experience. Part one's stories are in chronological order of occurrence, conveying the patient's experience. The moment shared may be during pregnancy, labor, delivery, or even some time after baby's death. In part two, the lesson from each story has been elaborated upon, with tangible strategies to follow when facing a similar situation. Both parts and all stories can be read consecutively, but it is not necessary.

For some, it was a challenge to pinpoint a moment where things went "right" when so many things had gone wrong. But, the purpose of this book is to share stories and strategies to help you do your best, so that future families can best heal. By sharing a brief glimpse of a health professional positively influencing an otherwise devastating time, the hope is that you will learn skills to bring to your daily practice.

Dear health professional, it is my intention to praise you through the stories that follow. I want you to feel encouraged and motivated to continue the work you do. I don't know if you are aware of the impact that you have on families when they are experiencing the worst moment of their lives. Your presence and interactions greatly affect a family not only in the moment that it's happening, but in the memories that are being created and referenced for the rest of their lives. That's a huge opportunity of blessing and also a large burden to bear. You play a tremendous role in a family's experience. You do amazing work every single time you face loss with your patient. You are the expert, even without personal experience, in how to navigate the most terrifying time of a parent's life. You guide them to do the unthinkable, to be present, to remain engaged, to create memories, to take photos, and to have experiences that they cannot relive in the future.

It is my observation and belief that if we can lessen a family's regret during this time, then the memories of their experience will help guide them positively in the future. When families receive support during time with their baby, whether in utero or after delivery, it enables the best chance at healing in their grief journey when they return home alone. With your direction and sensitivity, a family will leave the hospital (albeit without their baby) with memories that they would not have had, if not for your gentle guidance. All these moments that may seem insignificant to you, are their child's entire lifetime — their existence. Families replay these moments in their minds for the rest of their lives and your job is crucial in creating healing memories.

You are the first step in a life-long journey for families. You have an enormous job and I am so grateful for your willingness to learn from those who have generously shared sacred moments in this book. The way in which you care for your patients determines how a family experiences this loss. Your contribution is an integral part of their healing memories as parents. Your care, your human emotions, and your tender hand, helps heal a family from the very beginning.

So, thank you. You and your work are so appreciated, more than words can express.

OUR ONLY
Time

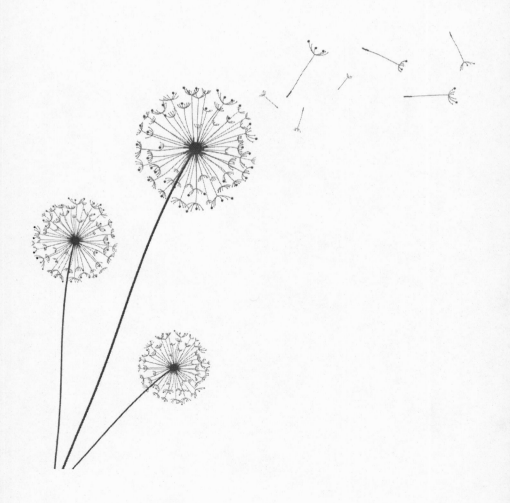

Introduction

OUR DAUGHTER, RUTHIE LOU, was born after a perfect pregnancy. Being pregnant was the best time in my life, as we imagined our growing family. However, upon birth, Ruthie Lou was not progressing as expected and our life was about to turn upside down. After two weeks in the NICU, it was learned that our daughter had a chromosomal abnormality requiring her to remain on life support for survival.

In those two weeks, we learned more about hospitals and medicine than I could have imagined. We had to make the agonizing decision to continue her life inevitably in the hospital or to remove life support. Ultimately, our hospital staff had the awareness of a freestanding pediatric palliative care facility and after removing her support, we had the privilege to transfer our family to George Mark Children's House. While it was predicted that she might only survive the night, Ruthie Lou lived another 12 days, the best days of our lives.

It was during those 33 days with our daughter, that we saw the true meaning of compassion and grace. The care that we received from nearly every doctor, nurse, social worker, child life therapist, and counselor was beyond what I knew existed. We were guided through the most painful time in our life as it transformed into beauty. The brief time that we had with Ruthie Lou was made peaceful solely because of the professionals who held our hands. Ruthie Lou's short days were filled with memories created and in a few short weeks, a lifetime was lived.

When we returned home without our beloved baby, our life had irreversibly changed. Not only did we have to make sense of how to move forward, we had to find out how to have a life worth living. Relationships that were created through Ruthie Lou's life felt like family, although I do realize the professionals were merely doing their

1

jobs. But, the memories of those days fueled us. They gave us hope and a belief that there was good in the world and if someone (or many someone's) could be our lifeline, then we could eventually do the same for others.

In considering how to best support parents, I truly believe it starts the moment that their life changes and it starts with you — the professional. When you positively impact parents during their moments of devastation, the hope is that when they enter the depths of grief at home, those memories will fuel them to continue living, to do their best in life, and maybe even be of support to someone else.

They say it takes a village to raise a child. It also takes a village to care for the parents who don't get to raise their child. You are that village; you are the first step in the healing of their hearts. This book was written lovingly in honor of you, for the work you do in the world and to educate those professionals wanting to do better.

Part One

STORIES OF PREGNANCY/INFANT LOSS

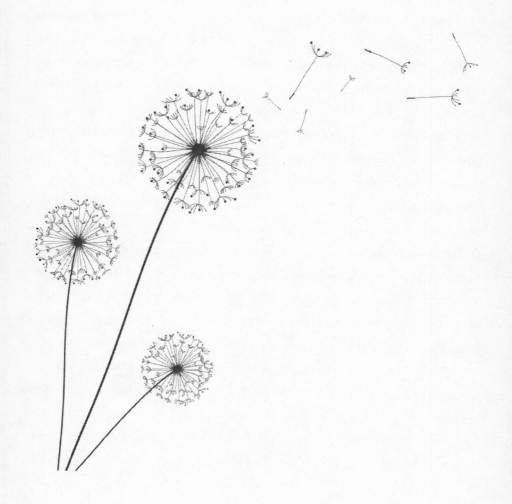

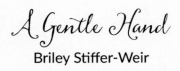

A Gentle Hand

Briley Stiffer-Weir

The pregnancy journey begins long before conception.

I can't breathe. The weight I feel on my chest is suffocating. There's a ringing in my ears and the quickly darkening room creates a tunnel of light through which I see only my husband sitting at the end. His look is one of worry and confusion. Our night out has suddenly been taken over by an oppressive cloud of fear and angst. It wasn't supposed to be this hard. People get pregnant every day — and even by accident! What if these fertility treatments don't work? With every fiber of my being, I am meant to be a mother and I am currently overwhelmed with this need and desire. I feel it as a heat in my chest and my heart beats more quickly, as my body goes weak.

It's as if there is a war within me — a battle between need and want. The man who sits across from me is the man of my dreams. I cannot picture a forever without him, and yet a life without children would be a sacrifice that I'm not certain I can handle. Over the course of several years, this loving man put himself through multiple surgeries to make our dreams come true. He loves me that much. Am I an awful person? Can I stifle the primal urge to mother in order to prove my love to him in return? Just maybe this last attempt will work, but what if it doesn't? What if it doesn't work!? The fear of defeat wins in the battle against hope tonight and we leave the restaurant before our meal arrives.

I wake from a sound sleep. A wave of panic is instantly upon me and envelops my body with its heat. I sweat and shake. I want these babies. I place two hands over my abdomen and try to calm myself and tuck my embryos in for the night as I listen to my husband sleeping beside me. Just breathe … Just stay positive. I cry myself to sleep like so many nights before.

I go to work at the clinic as a perinatal and infertility nurse coordinator. I wear a smile that's authentic and unforced. The care and compassion I give my patients is genuine and I know that I positively impact their experiences. I help navigate their pregnancies, their deliveries, their struggles, and their experiences of loss. I support them, grieve with them, and offer an empathetic ear when they feel concerned. I'm told that my words of advice and encouragement are helpful and some of the best they've received. And yet, every day, I feel alone in my own fears and struggles. I turn inward, feeling isolated. The words I tell others do little to comfort my own fear of loss. Will I get the life I long for?

I wake in the middle of the night in excruciating pain. Something is wrong. Again, I place two hands over my abdomen and breathe deeply. I try to picture this treatment being successful and growing into a healthy pregnancy, but the pain cuts through my thoughts …

I arrive the next morning at work — diaphoretic, pale, and in agony. My doctor, whom is both my employer and my friend, notices immediately and ushers me into an exam room. My blood pressure is 170/118 with a high pulse. Beads of sweat fall down my back and forehead as I explain the course of the night. An ultrasound reveals ovarian hyperstimulation syndrome resulting from the in vitro, with free fluid in my pelvis and abdomen caused by the bursting follicles.

"Will this hurt my chances of success," I cry.

"We'll have to see, my dear," my doctor tenderly replies.

I call the infertility doctor and I'm told to drink Gatorade and that I'll "be fine." My pain is not addressed. My questions go unanswered. The severity of my case gets placed amongst all the other untoward side effects and I am treated like a statistic. My OBGYN gets on the phone and explains his concerns. He, too, is placated.

My doctor sees my pain, has seen the ultrasound, as well as my worrisome vital signs. He wants to admit me to the hospital immediately, but I am stubborn and scared. Scared of the financial burden and that the medications may affect my chances of success. He's worried — I can see it in the lines of his face. We reach a compromise and hurry to the hospital for some supplies.

Minutes later, he walks me into a room where he's made a bed atop our DEXA machine. I'm tucked in and he starts an IV with fluids and gives me pain medication that he picked up for me at the pharmacy. Each hour, he personally checks in on me and reevaluates my vitals and my pain. He does this for eight hours, even after the office has closed. His words of comfort are scarce, but his presence is calming and supportive.

"Dr. Stokes, I'm so scared I won't get these babies!"

He lays a gentle hand of my shoulder and his eyes connect with mine.

"I know my dear. I'm here."

From Infertility to Empowerment

Rachel McGrath

Allow mom to be an active participant in her medical care. Listen to her.

Infertility and pregnancy loss was something I never expected to experience, and quite frankly, I didn't realize just how many women around the world faced such challenges until I was going through it myself. As a woman who was always determined to have a family, like many others in my situation, I didn't start until my late thirties. This wasn't through lack of want, but for me, I hadn't found and married my 'Mr. Right' until I was 35. You can't hurry love ...

We took several months to conceive our first baby, and when we finally saw that positive pregnancy test, we were over the moon. Sadly, and very unexpectedly, however, we lost that pregnancy, with a scan showing no heartbeat at 10 weeks. I went on to have three further pregnancies, each ending in the first trimester, and each time I was struggling to find answers to help me understand why this was happening. The common reason I was given was my age. However, there was no proof or basis to this diagnosis, except the basic assumption that my "eggs were old and, therefore, impacting the ability for my pregnancies to progress."

Initially, the doctors and nurses I had contact with seemed non-committed to my desire to become a mum. My age was the excuse not to pursue other tests, and I had a very bad experience with a D&C (dilation and curettage) procedure to remove my fourth pregnancy that left me with further damage to my uterine lining. Consequently, this caused me even further issues in getting pregnant. For some time, I felt that the doctors and medical staff I had been dealing with were only treating me like a number, not a patient. I didn't feel anyone was taking my case seriously, and I had limited confidence that I would be able to start a family without taking back some control.

I didn't give up.

After several incidents where I felt pushed aside, or where I felt the doctors and nurses at my local surgery and the hospital were treating my plight for a baby like a trivial case, I decided to take my case into my own hands.

I changed doctors and requested the support of a specific specialist who could help me with my fertility obstacles. It was now over two years into my pregnancy journey and I finally felt that I was getting the attention to my situation that I had longed for. The doctor at my local surgery sat me down and explained my options, including surrogacy or adoption if I couldn't conceive. They gave me advice on counseling and directed me to information that might help me understand the grief and frustration I was feeling. The specialist I sought after conducted a thorough examination of my uterus and diagnosed my condition quickly. He was honest, transparent, and direct. He explained that I had a protein S deficiency (sticky blood) that meant my blood was thick and clotting, causing those four pregnancies to fail in the early stages. He also diagnosed me with Asherman syndrome (a uterine condition) as a result of the D&C procedure, which was now impacting my ability to conceive. We had a plan, and whilst he could not promise me a baby, he assured me he would do his best to increase my chances. For the first time in almost three years I felt supported and informed.

After three surgeries to correct the damage within my uterus, I was finally told that my body was ovulating and undergoing a full cycle: it was ready to start a process of conception again. I felt overjoyed and hopeful. The specialist also gave me assurance that in the event of a pregnancy, there was a plan to treat my protein S deficiency, to hopefully prevent any further miscarriages. As I look back at the eight months of treatment I underwent, I felt reassured that I was in good hands no matter what.

The good news is that I did fall pregnant, just four months after that last surgical procedure. Immediately, I was transferred back to my general doctor with a plan and medications to manage my condition and give my pregnancy the best care possible. My doctor gave me options about my care throughout the pregnancy. I was allocated a new hospital (different than the one where I had experienced my losses) and was assured that I would be frequently scanned and checked upon to ensure that the pregnancy had its best chance of succeeding. I finally felt relaxed about the medical care I was given, and the doctors and nurses at the hospital were responsive and empathetic to my case.

My pregnancy was marked as high risk and I had monthly check-ups and regular scans to ensure that my baby was on track and monitored for any anomalies. I was never put on hold and I never had to wait to be seen when things were worrying me. I was supported without question through the entire pregnancy.

I had choices, too, and I felt empowered to make decisions that were right for both my baby and me. When my son was born, I was overjoyed, and I received heartfelt congratulations from the medical staff and my specialist for the journey I had travelled awaiting the arrival of our healthy and happy baby. The journey to a healthy pregnancy and carrying my son to term had been tumultuous, but I cannot fault the level of care I received. Once I made the decision to change medical care, I never looked back.

I had two very different experiences with my doctors and the medical profession throughout my fertility journey, which reinforced to me that as a patient, we should question, challenge, and push for the best care possible. We deserve the best care and fertility is a growing issue. The more empathy and awareness the medical profession can bring, the more likely it is that women will be supported to find the right solution, helping them to achieve their goal of parenthood.

This is Our Baby

Angela Olsen

All losses, no matter gestation or age of baby, are worthy of validation.
Validate all losses.

After 13 months of trying to conceive, there it was. I held in my hand the result that said I was going to be a momma. Bliss. Joy. Excitement. It was 4:30 in the morning and I quickly went upstairs to wake up my husband to tell him what the little stick had just told me — we were going to be parents! In an instant, we had planned out the next 18 years: boy or girl, what their personality would be like, how tall would they be, and so on and so forth.

I quickly called my best friend who was still sleeping. After numerous missed calls, she finally answered. I said, "Good morning, auntie Carolyn." She didn't understand why I was calling her so early in the morning. Referring to her as auntie only added to her confusion. I repeated myself, twice, until she finally understood what I meant. She couldn't have been any happier for us.

When I was five weeks along, we decided to share with our family that we were expecting, and after that, we told everyone else. Why not? We were on cloud nine and wanted the world to know. Soon after we made our announcement, we had an ultrasound done. We could actually see our baby's heartbeat fluttering on the monitor. He or she was perfect already and getting to see this only solidified our love even more. I downloaded an app on my phone to track the baby's development; each week brought new and exciting changes.

One day while I was at work, I went to the bathroom. After wiping, I noticed a faint brownish/reddish residue on my toilet paper. Never in those first moments did we even think about losing our baby. My emotions overtook me. Fear. Panic. Dread.

Thankfully I work with my doctor, so I walked over to his office. My heart was pounding and my stomach was uneasy. I explained what happened and he asked if I had any cramping and if I felt pregnant. My reply was quick, "Yes I feel pregnant, and no I haven't had any cramping." He gave me reassurance and encouraged me to rest and watch for bleeding, explaining that it can be very common for women to have spotting during pregnancy. For the rest of the day, I kept second-guessing myself if I actually felt pregnant or not. At this point, I was 10 weeks along and pretty sure everything I had felt up until this point was pregnancy related. Still, the uneasy feeling in my stomach lingered and so did the spotting.

The following day, I asked to have an ultrasound because I just couldn't shake the feeling that something wasn't right. It was a drizzly cold day and my husband drove us to the hospital. We were both lost in our own thoughts, not speaking much and both hoping that everything would turn out okay.

Once we arrived, the usually chatty ultrasound technician was particularly quiet, not speaking as openly as she had done during our first visit with her. The longer the exam took, my sadness grew. Slowly, I began to cry. I turned my head from the screen, not sure at all of what I was looking at anyway. I saw my husband's face; he, too, had watery eyes, but we held our hands tightly together. At the end of the exam, she told us that the doctor would be getting in touch with us soon with the results and that she hoped to see us again soon.

We left the hospital and sat in our car in the parking lot. We turned the radio down low and just sat there, not sure exactly what to do or where to go. I felt numb.

Shortly after, my phone rang. I could see it was my doctor, but I didn't want to answer because I knew what he was going to tell me. I put it on speaker phone.

"Angela, I am so sorry to tell you this, but your baby has died."

That sentence broke me. I sobbed "no" over and over again. I didn't want to believe it. My doctor told me to come into the office since we were in the parking lot. We ended the call and my husband and I fell into each other's arms and cried. There was a comfort in knowing that he was hurting as much as I was, and that we would go through this hell together.

We held each other for a long time before we composed ourselves enough to walk into the office where I worked. We went through the back door because I didn't want to see anybody. My doctor opened the door and led us into the exam room. My eyes and face were already red and swollen from crying.

My doctor gave me the biggest hug and continued to apologize for the loss of our baby. He explained that in the ultrasound the baby had died shortly after six weeks, but my body had not yet released anything, even after four weeks. This is something called a missed miscarriage. He was gentle, caring, and supportive and answered the few questions that we had. He continued to validate the life I had carried, even for the short period of time it was, and that he was sorry for our loss.

Any pregnancy loss, no matter how far along one may be, is still a tremendous loss to parents. You're not "only" four, six, nine weeks along, assuming that will make it easier on your heart. This was our first baby and I will forever hold him or her in my heart. My doctor validated and acknowledged our baby. He acknowledged that our baby was real and, likewise, our loss was real.

True Empathy

Jessica McCoy

Discovering a life-limiting or fatal prenatal diagnosis is life changing.
Support families in their grief.

As I lay on the exam table with my legs in the air, I felt so vulnerable and so unprepared for what was about to happen. I had talked myself through it before. I was counseled. I prayed. I had said goodbye to Evie. But, nothing can prepare you for the real goodbye. Ending a wanted pregnancy is something I wouldn't wish upon my worst enemy, if I ever had one. And yet, here I was, saying goodbye to my little girl before we even got to meet — on the outside anyway. Our souls had known each other for nearly six months at that point. I knew her awake times. What food she liked and what food she really didn't like. I knew what music made her dance and that when I laughed really hard, she would wake up and start kicking. I knew the shape of her beautiful lips. I saw them on the ultrasound before I also saw that her spine bubbled out of her back. Before I knew she also had a chromosomal deletion. I knew her before I knew what was wrong with her. I knew she didn't deserve to suffer. I knew I loved her with all of my being, with everything in me.

The exam table was cold. My whole body shivered, teeth chattering. A nurse came in. She had scrubs on and a blue surgical cap. She said, "Hi, I'm Jenny and I'm here for you. If you want me to hold your hand, I am here for you, whatever you need." She was young and so very pretty, with a hoop nose ring. She had such kind eyes. The ultrasound tech put the transducer on my belly and once they found Evie's heart, the doctor put a needle into my belly and stopped her heart. I started sobbing and Jenny held my hand. My whole body shook with grief. I looked up at Jenny and she had tears in her eyes. I remember wondering if she always teared up, or if she was just so moved because I so obviously wanted my baby. And then I knew. I knew she recognized that Evie was real. That Evie's life deserved to be grieved.

As the doctor was sticking the laminaria sticks into my cervix, I looked at Jenny, wide-eyed. I didn't know it would hurt so badly. I sobbed even harder, and cried out, "Oh, nooo … Nooo … Evie." Jenny held my hand as I squeezed hard, transferring some of my pain to her. Once the sticks were inserted, I just sobbed on the table while Jenny and the doctor tried to help me up. The doctor then told me they were so very sorry for my loss and left the room.

With tears still in her eyes, Jenny hugged me. As she touched her hand to her heart, she told me it was an honor for her to be here for me and that she was so, so sorry. Another nurse came in to wheel me back into the room where my husband was waiting. I sobbed for Evie. I sobbed for what could have been. For what should have been. I also sobbed because of Jenny's kindness and for her true empathy for me. I could tell that she was changed that day. My experience moved her in some way. I felt it.

Jenny recognized that Evie was a person. That Evie was loved. Jenny was aware how completely broken I was, having to say goodbye to my daughter. She knew that my loss was deep and that Evie deserved to be grieved. In that space I was allowed to feel the enormity of my loss. On the cold exam table, I was given the space to begin to grieve the death of my daughter, and it was exactly what I needed.

Knowing Your Role

Heather Browne

Help navigate medical processes. Advocate for families no matter their decision.

"I don't want to lie to you and tell you everything looks okay," said the ultrasound technician. This was the first sign of any complication.

21 weeks, two days pregnant

Days before, my husband and I joked this would be an "uneventful, uninformative (anatomy) ultrasound." We were sticking to our decision not to find out if we were having a third boy or our first girl. We wanted a surprise.

"I'm going to get the doctor." My husband and I were left alone in a dark room. This wasn't the surprise we were looking for.

I turned to my husband, "Do you think it's something really bad?"

We were moved to another room where we paced, waiting — too nervous to sit. The moment hung in the stale air a little longer than the clock registered.

And then this, "Your baby has spina bifida. There's a hole in the spine."

Though my doctor was direct, my mind wandered to a colleague who has a daughter with spina bifida. Okay, my baby's life will be like hers, I thought, as if everyone diagnosed with a disorder suffers the same level of severity. When I refocused on the present conversation, my doctor seemed to be apologizing for an inevitable loss. "Wait a minute," I asked. "Are you telling me this is a reason people have an abortion?" I was bitter and naïve. My doctor, recognizing my ignorance, shared the high percentage of pregnancies terminated as a result of spina bifida.

What is wrong with those mothers? How could they not want their (special needs) baby? Surely, abortions were only for unwanted babies. I judged other women — other mothers — not imagining their reality could be mine.

We left, awaiting a call from a specialist, desperate for information, but wary of online research. We agreed to gather our knowledge from my colleague and our doctors, exclusively.

Calling my coworker to share this intimate information felt foreign in my head, but certain in my heart. She openly shared her experience with the rapid escalation of doctors and questions she wished she had asked. The next day, she flagged pages in her spina bifida book for our basic understanding. This was my reality check. For the first time, this was actually happening. To me. To us. To our baby.

21 weeks, three days pregnant

I awoke with an intense maternal instinct to advocate for our baby. I bought a journal to record and organize the barrage of information — a place to put the noise in my head so that my mind could clearly receive additional information.

The local perinatal diagnostic center called, and my husband and I were rushed in for another ultrasound where the maternal-fetal medicine doctor, Sarah, led with, "Heather, we need to do an amniocentesis and a prenatal chromosomal microarray analysis immediately." Her hyper-focus on our baby clearly communicated the severity of our needs.

After the procedure, Sarah had better visibility of our child's spine. Her best professional estimate of the level of the lesion: "S4, maybe S5."

Okay, my friend's daughter is S4. We're okay.

And then, Sarah inquired, "Are you two serious about exploring options for keeping this baby?"

"Absolutely," we responded in unison.

Sarah explained the urgency of timing and the need for travel to the top fetal spina bifida hospital in the country, several states away.

At that point, we reduced our contact with the world to fewer than ten people. My husband and I arranged to be away from work and our living children. We packed a bag and left home, racing an impending snowstorm. From the car, I called my best friend; the children's hospital is near her, and we would need a place to stay.

Between the physical commotion of being shuffled from place to place and the clamoring voices in my head, I craved stillness and silence. A teacher by trade, facts provide me clarity and peace, whereas opinions and anomalies clutter my thoughts. We used the car ride to investigate a few credible websites and learn about life expectancy and quality of life. We talked about sacrifices and empowered each other to hear a detailed prognosis. We finished our drive in the dark, wondering and waiting.

21 weeks, four days – 22 weeks pregnant

For four days, we were snowed in at my best friend's house, just 15 miles away from our only hope. We worked the phones for appointments. We planned for potential financial obligations with our insurance company. We missed our children's hugs. We lived a reoccurring nightmare — trying to run toward something with our legs paralyzed, stuck in molasses. Four long, excruciating days with our life on pause.

22 weeks, one day pregnant

Finally, it was appointment day! I craved the fast pace and urgency of care we had previously experienced. Momentum felt like progress. I braced myself … and …

We waited. We waited for paperwork, hospital administrators, an ultrasound, fetal MRI, fetal echocardiogram, genetic counselor, pediatric neurosurgeon, director of obstetrical services. Most importantly, we waited for answers. The silence was deafening.

Finally, we squeezed into a tight room with a panel of fetal spina bifida surgeons for the official diagnosis: "With 100% certainty … L2." This was far worse than Dr. Sarah predicted.

L2 meant clubfoot deformity, loss of sexual function, bowel and bladder incontinence, scoliosis, renal failure, kidney infections, urinary stasis and reflux, posterior fossa compression syndrome, Chiari II hindbrain herniation, hydrocephaly, shunts — an endless list. Even with fetal surgery, no one could give our child a quality of life that fit our definition of humane. We needed to process.

22 weeks, two days pregnant

First appointment of the day: Over an hour listening to a perinatal advance practice nurse detailing every risk of fetal surgery for just me. The next hour, she shared the implications of fetal surgery for our unborn baby. For the first time, this level of detail, while necessary, was overwhelming.

We had our answer. We had clarity.

The only way we felt we could protect our baby was to take on the inevitable pain and suffering ourselves. It would have been easy to continue with our itinerary for the day, but the most difficult words we ever said aloud were, "I think we need to explore abortion."

Our judgment-free nurse coordinator immediately shifted gears and found a doctor to explain what our new path entailed. Thankfully, she didn't condemn me the way I condemned others seven days ago. Instead, she comforted us, saying, "I think you'd be crazy not to consider abortion."

Within minutes, that doctor put us in touch with a trusted OB-GYN's office (a personal friend of hers who would perform the procedure expediently and empathetically). We called his office right away to schedule our consultation for the next morning — no more waiting.

Before leaving the children's hospital, we met with a child life specialist who asked us about our spirituality, our families, and the personalities of our two sons. She provided us a framework for sharing our story that honored our wishes and children's books to read with our boys to explain the loss simply, honestly, and concretely. We asked only one request of her — could she please find out if our baby was a boy or a girl?

Hours later, sitting in a parked car, we opened the sealed envelope to reveal three little letters: b-o-y. A third boy. The boy that would complete our family. The boy we'd never meet, never hold, never kiss.

We decided to give him a name that conveyed our resounding feeling from this experience: Ace, meaning oneness and unity. Ace strengthened our marriage. Ace embodied the collective health care professionals who delivered us to our answer. Ace symbolized the unity of our extended families who came together to care for our children and us.

Everyone in our process played their role seamlessly. We didn't need our family to offer their opinions on spina bifida or ending a wanted pregnancy — that was our doctors' role. We didn't need our friends to question our every move — that was our role as Ace's parents. And we didn't need our doctors to soften the blow — that was our family's role. With each person playing their respective part, we were able to fulfill our role as parents without a single moment of regret, without any unanswered questions. We have clarity. We have peace. We have unity. We have Ace.

Making a Choice

Stacey Porter

Inform parents of all options. Support their decision.

My two previous pregnancies had been picture perfect, but when I was pregnant with our third, it turned into a guessing game. Doctors would find one thing to keep an eye on and by the next month's appointment, whatever it had been had resolved, but there was something new that would trigger caution. Eventually, I went on to develop severe preeclampsia. At 24 weeks, 5 days, my condition had declined enough that my primary OB recommended that I be transferred to another hospital 1.5 hours away because they were better equipped to care for micro-preemies. After an anxiety filled ambulance ride, I settled into a room at the new hospital and baby and I continued to be constantly monitored. My most vivid memory of that day was when my husband and I were given an impossible choice.

I was still being monitored for my rising protein levels and elevated blood pressure. Back at our home hospital, they had prepared me for an early delivery by making sure baby got the first dose of a medication that would help to mature the lungs. They told me that I would need another dose at the other hospital.

I had only been there for about three hours when the maternal fetal medicine doctor checked in with my husband and me. He said he'd been watching the progress with me and baby for a while and that he was concerned. It looked like baby was having decelerations in the heartbeat, which were becoming more frequent. It was at this point that he told us that it was 100% up to us, but that what he was seeing was indicating that things were going to continue to decline for the baby and me. When he talked with us, he sat down and spoke in a tone that was not alarming, not distant, not matter-of-fact, not authoritarian, but instead was warm, genuinely compassionate, and not at all hurried. He spoke to us as parents and people whose world had been turned upside down already and was about to tilt to a completely alternate axis.

We spoke about the options: 1) We could choose to keep baby in utero for as long as possible, but when things went south (and all signs were indicating that they would) they would need to act quickly to do whatever needed to be done at that time. 2) We could choose to exert a little more control over the situation and schedule a C-section delivery for that evening. He also offered to have a neonatologist come up to speak with us, which we were more than happy to take him up on.

When the neonatologist arrived, he doubled checked that we understood what was going on, and then I asked the question no mother or father ever wants to ask, but desperately needs to know: "What are the chances of survival for our baby this early?" The answer he gave was truthful and caring, but it still sliced through me like the sharpest blade there ever was. "At your baby's age, they are still very small and not able to regulate very well outside the womb. We will do everything we can, but chance of survival for a baby at this age is less than 40%".

How could they ask me, ask us, to make this choice? I wasn't mad at them; both these doctors had been super understanding and took time to talk, asked if we had questions. But, the only words I heard played like a record in my head, "less than 40%". Less than half. They made sure we had the information we needed and took their leave for us to think about this choice. The maternal fetal doctor came back after we'd had some time to process and we had a very helpful conversation about how what he was seeing in my stats indicated that even if we chose to let baby stay in utero, it was very unlikely that it would be long enough to make a true difference in chances of survival. That was telling at a time when even a few days to a week made a huge impact in baby's development and survival.

The baby's decelerations in heart rate were showing increasing distress. In my mind, our choice, my choice, was to be a "bad mother" by letting our baby stay in utero, where it wasn't even really safe anymore, and to allow potentially fatal things to happen for either baby or me, or both of us. Or, to be a "bad mother" and force our child out into a world that he or she was not ready for with dangerously low odds. The doctors did not push us to make a quick decision, and they did not force us in either direction, which helped to empower us as the decision makers for our child — even though it was one that I wished anyone else would be the one to make at the time. We felt supported and informed. Both doctors made it a point to reassure us that they would do everything in their power to help give the best outcome for me and our baby, whichever path we chose.

Taking all the information into consideration, my husband and I made the best decision we could at the time: to bring the baby into the world by controlling what we could, to ensure the best chance of survival by allowing everyone to be prepared for a C-section. We weren't prepared to meet our baby that day. We didn't even know if we were having a boy or a girl. We already had a 4-year-old son and 3-year-old daughter, so we had figured we would allow the gender of this baby to be a surprise … This was not the surprise we were expecting at all. I swallowed back the lump in my throat and blinked through tears and said to my husband, "I guess we better pick out some names."

She Shared My Grief

Adrien McGoon

Having an emotional response is human. It's okay to show your emotions.

During a routine appointment at 27 weeks, my husband and I learned that our son had passed. Suddenly, everything became a heartbreaking blur of pain and sadness. I assumed that the doctors and nurses handled losses like mine routinely and that it was just another workday, but I soon discovered that it was not.

As I was laboring, the staff was very kind and considerate. My emotions were like a roller coaster; one minute I'd be okay, the next a sobbing mess, followed by anger and confusion.

My mom and my husband stayed with me pretty much the entire time I was in the hospital. During the second day, we were sitting and talking, eating lunch, and my mind wandered away from where I was and why I was there. Then, like a tidal wave, it hit me, the future I had imagined with our son that would no longer be happening and I began to weep. A social worker came into our room at one point and shared that losing a baby is especially hard because you're not losing the memory of a person that lived but rather a future that you hoped to have with them, losing the memories you had hoped to share.

When it came time to deliver, a doctor and a nurse named Anne attended to me. When my son Henry entered the world, a great sadness filled the room. Not only were my husband and I crying, but Anne was also weeping with us. I didn't expect it, but it truly meant a lot to me. It was a very welcome surprise to see that she, too, shared in my grief and that my loss mattered to her, too.

Henry was much smaller than what I had imagined he would be, but he was so perfect. My husband, my mom, and my mother-in-law were all present when he arrived and we each took a turn holding him. I tried to take in every inch of him: looking at how long his tiny fingers were, at his sweet little mouth, and his toes that looked like mine. We took pictures of him and with him to remember him by and when we felt it was time, we asked the nurse to come take him.

The nursing staff also took pictures of Henry, and presented them to us in a memory box with other keepsakes. Inside the box was a tiny outfit that they had tried to put Henry in, but it was too big, a print of his hand and foot, and a tiny blanket he had been wrapped in. The box now sits in our bedroom on a shelf and every once in awhile, I will sit down and look in it. I'm not sure that there will ever be a time that I don't cry when I do.

It isn't every day that babies die in hospitals. It isn't routine. Anne's tears showed me that she cared, that she, too, was sad and that it was okay to cry, to grieve. Her emotional response let me know that losing Henry wasn't routine. I'll never forget that moment. I cherish it. It changed me. In that moment, I knew the staff would take care of my sweet baby boy and he would always be remembered.

Allowing Time

Blandine de Coincy

Slow down. Breathe. Allow the family time to process the magnitude of their loss. There is no rush.

This story is about my baby girl, Sixtine, born still at 40 weeks. But, more so, it is about Muriel, our midwife. She was there from the very beginning until the end. We would not have made it without her.

We met Muriel when I wanted to have a home birth for our first pregnancy, but my husband had disagreed. We looked for a place where it could be just like home, but with all the necessities of the hospital to appease my husband.

We fell in love with Muriel because she was all we wanted and all we were looking for; she was smart, experienced, funny, and never stressed (or it didn't show). Muriel would get straight to the point without over-analyzing things, which made everything feel simple and easy.

One morning, I had a vision. My husband and I were in a church with a tiny white coffin. It made me cry and feel so worried, but I assumed it was only pregnancy hormones. But, later that night, when I could not remember when I had last felt my baby move, I called Muriel.

We decided to meet at the clinic in Paris.

Muriel hooked me to the fetal monitor and got a heartbeat. At first, it looked like the baby's, but because I was so stressed, it was actually mine that was being heard. Later, the OB-GYN walked in with the sonogram and told me, "It's over."

He wanted me to deliver the baby right away, but I said no. I had just learned my baby was gone; I was not prepared to go into labor and meet my stillborn child.

I was so appreciative of my midwife being in charge. I was not ready and she gave me time. She let us do what we felt was right for us. We went downstairs and had a smoke. We walked in Paris for a long time that night. She let me run my own agenda.

The next morning, I was ready. I felt like a walking grave and needed this baby to come out. I called Muriel and she discovered I didn't have to be induced because I was already in labor. And, because Muriel respected my wishes and let me have time to become psychologically prepared (as much as we could in this terrible situation), I had a smooth delivery.

Muriel handed the baby to us. It was both the hardest and the most beautiful time of our lives. She was a girl. She was so beautiful, so perfect … But stillborn.

We were not able to function. We were in such a blur. Muriel helped us to put a diaper on her, dress her. She took pictures and handprints. We cherish all these treasures that she thought about for us.

We spent many hours with our Sixtine. I held her, kissed her, touched her, and looked at her everywhere and at every angle. It was our only time.

Then, Muriel wrapped her in a blanket and took her to the mortuary room. She was always respectful of us and of Sixtine, of her tiny body. Every time we would see our baby, she would have her prepared in a baby bassinet; we never saw her as she was at the mortuary.

We gave Muriel's cellphone number to the funeral home, and both of them arranged the care of our baby. It made things easier. On the morning Sixtine was laid to rest, Muriel was there, too. She was the one who put Sixtine in her coffin. She was the very first one who held her, and the very last one too. She drove in the car with us and with the coffin. She was there at church for the ceremony. She was there at the cemetery for our last goodbye. Having Muriel with us and available at all times made this terrible journey easier.

We were blessed and lucky enough to have three beautiful and healthy children after Sixtine. Muriel was the one and only who helped me give birth to all of our five children; four who can run, one who can fly. And, for all of that, we will never be thankful enough.

Merci, Muriel.

He is Safe Now

Lindsay Gibson

Acknowledge a birthing mother. Create a safe space for her to deliver her baby.

"Your son is safe now, Lindsay. My job is to make sure you are safe, too." I looked up at her face and stared into her eyes that looked so soft and safe in that one moment. Those are the words I needed to hear in my nightmare. I actually felt safe and supported in her capable hands. I squinted against the blinding operating room lights that sparkled behind her head and reflected through my tears. Fresh new tears had welled up and poured down my face, washing over the old ones in my swollen eyelids.

"I love you, Joseph. Mommy is so sorry," I whispered, as everything went black. When I woke up, my husband, Jason, was lying beside me in the cramped hospital bed. I was in the recovery room, and he was wiping up the sweat on my face with a towel. My heart pounded against my body that was shaking uncontrollably. Then I remembered and reached down to feel my soft belly that was once pregnant with my precious baby. His little body was gone.

"No. No. No, Jason, no!" I sobbed against his strong chest. The surgeon's last words rang in my mind. Your son is safe now.

It had been an entire week in the hospital since the day we found out that our sweet boy had died and I would give birth to a stillborn. What was supposed to be a routine check turned into the worst day of our life. Only hours before on that day, I had felt his strong kicks, reminding me to stay strong and that we would soon be together. His kicks were my reassurance that everything was okay, despite the debilitating hyperemesis gravidarum that I had been fighting the entire pregnancy. These daily kicks helped me to know that he was safe, no matter how sick I was. Yet, when those kicks were suddenly not there anymore, I was urged to head the hospital the next day.

For the next four days, medical professionals surrounded me. They never acknowledged me as a birthing mother. Despite the fact that he was gone, I was still birthing him. Only in the end, did a kind surgeon tell me that even though he had passed away, he was still safe. As a stillbirth mom, this was what I needed to hear. But it was too late. After four days of trying to birth him, and despite all attempts by my obstetrician, my body would not let him go. As a result, he had to be surgically removed.

As Jason began to calm my sobs and still my body, I began to relax, feeling myself ease into the safety he created on the bed. Why couldn't I release him? The week was replaying in my mind at such a fast speed, as I desperately tried to make sense of what just happened.

On the first day that we were admitted in the hospital, my pastor came. She prayed with me, listened, held my hand, and by the third day of labor with Joseph, she saw what was happening and what I needed to hear. In the privacy of my room, she took my hand, "Talk to him Lindsay. He is still with you. And now talk to your body, tell it that it is safe and to let him go." I could barely comprehend her words and all I could do was cry. I held protectively to my womb and felt powerless against the 26 weeks that I held him safe inside of me. The mother-baby bond was strong and I loved this little one so much. Sensing what was on my mind, she continued, "He loves you, too. You are still his mommy. But you need to let his body go now. It is safe to do that here."

Within minutes after her departure, my doctor came in trying to figure out what "drug" to give me next, visibly frustrated with how slow things were progressing. I calmly told her to please stop upping the drugs and that I wanted time to release him myself. What she said next will forever stay in my mind, "Why? Let me just do my job. It's not like these drugs will hurt it because the fetus is dead."

The fetus? Dead? What my pastor encouraged me to do was shattered by her harsh words. I felt no support or safety as a birthing mother. Whether my baby was alive or stillborn, I needed to birth him and let my own body do it without fear. The hospital team failed to give me what I needed most: encouragement, compassion, and the support to be a brave birthing mama.

My son was gone here on earth, but I was still his mom. He was still with me and always would be. And, most importantly in that moment, I needed it to be known that I was still giving birth. Doctors and nurses had been in and out, scratching their heads as to why it was taking so long, counting the days, and continuously loading me up on all kinds of drugs. I felt like a medical experiment instead of a mom giving birth. While their intentions may have been good, no one recognized my overwhelming grief and desire to not be drugged and be present for this important birth.

I hold no bitterness towards my birth workers, because forgiveness is an important part of healing. Instead, what my pastor shared with me that day is what I wish they knew. It was first and foremost a birth. I had a deep need to feel supported in my choices along the way. Birthing him was healing for me, not something to be drugged or treated as a procedure. My son, not a fetus, was and is a special part of my life to this day. Finally, I also needed to recognize that grief was not the enemy for me. I needed to feel my sadness and make space for it in the birthing experience. Making space for grief has been the path to healing and finding my joy again. Even though, I left with empty arms, my heart continues to be full of love.

They Saw My Baby

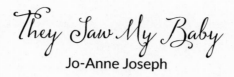

Jo-Anne Joseph

Show compassion in your words and actions. Remember that this is a loved and wanted child.

I lay on the hospital bed hooked up to a portable sonar machine, extremely anxious and just wanting to hear the words, "Everything is okay". It was my third check-up in a month. The doctor entered my room, barely introducing himself and proceeded to move the probe over my very pregnant belly. His face dropped slightly and he moved the probe around a bit more. He sighed and looked at me.

"I am sorry, but your baby has passed away. There is no heartbeat," he said.

Those words altered my life. I stopped breathing for a few seconds and I looked at him with the most confused expression on my face. I looked at the doctor, whose name I didn't quite catch. He was a stranger to me and I flinched as he placed his cold hand on mine. He handed me the copy of the ultrasound pictures, which I held close. What was he sorry for? Surely this was a mistake.

"I don't know why these things happen, Mrs. Joseph. Dr. D will be here soon, just rest. I'll be in to check on you in a bit."

"Are you sure? What happened?" I asked.

"We'll have to do some tests, but only once the baby is delivered," he said.

I didn't say anything else, just nodded, barely hearing him anymore because there was nothing more to say. My baby was gone. I cannot recall whether he returned. I made the heartbreaking calls to family members and I sat in the hospital room crying alone, waiting for my husband to arrive, waiting to tell him that our baby was gone. A few nurses came in and out of my room; none of them seemed to acknowledge the fact that my baby had died. I was prepped for surgery; today was the day my baby would be born and yet, for them, they were there to do a job.

The room felt cold and even the winter sun streaming in through the windows brought me no comfort. There would be no comfort, not anymore. Silent tears streamed down my cheeks and wrapped themselves around my face; they fell onto my pillow and ran into my mouth while I waited for what seemed like an eternity for my husband to join me. To join me in my disbelief, join me in my sadness, and join me in my heartache. One of the more senior nurses came into the room and said she was sorry. I remember nodding briefly and smiling at her feebly, then resuming my initial position, staring at the wall beside the window.

A few hours later, after some time with my husband and other family members, I was lying on my hospital bed in the foyer outside the surgery room waiting for my husband. The tears didn't fall; I just stared at the ceiling, wanting it to fall on me, wanting to wake up from this awful nightmare. I felt a hand rest gently on mine. I saw that it was Dr. D, my obstetrician. She'd arrived, and even in my sadness, I was glad to see her. She was familiar to me; she knew me, she knew my family, and she knew my baby.

"Hi Rehka," she said softly. "I'm so sorry." She took my hand in hers and we stood like that for a while. She glanced away, but not before I saw the tears glaze over her eyes. She wiped them away and was still holding my hand when the anesthetist arrived. Unlike the other doctor, I knew that Dr. D was sorry, I could feel it. It radiated off her. Babies aren't supposed to die. No, they're supposed to live and grow and feel love. When my husband arrived, we went in, to our fate, to the inevitable. A half an hour later she handed our baby to us, but there was only silence. I glanced down at my daughter and the tears slipped down my cheeks. My husband held me.

"It's a girl," she said. "She really is a girl." Her voice trailed off and broke. She stepped away. To many it would not have been a remarkable thing to say, but to me, it was everything. She remembered me, she remembered us, and she remembered the numerous scans we had to take before we inconclusively agreed we were having a girl. She was the kind doctor who laughed with me when my three-year-old started crying when he found out he was having a sister instead of a brother.

"What is her name," the anesthetist asked.

"Zia Sarai," I said, just above a whisper.

"That's a beautiful name, Mrs. Joseph," she said, smiling.

Four years later, I realize that on that day, my doctor and anesthetist did something amazing. They saw my baby as just that, a baby, not just a third trimester loss. They asked her name and showed humanity and compassion. Dr. D was not too professional to show her sadness. For the longest time, I'd forgotten how much comfort I'd felt, despite the heaviness and sadness that surrounded me, mostly because the overall experience in hospital was not the most pleasant one. It was easy to forget that anyone was kind or good to us. Oblivious to our experience, I had a pathologist come in and ask me to consent for bloods to be taken from my baby and a nurse tell me that it was time to feed my baby. But now, I remember Dr. D and her anesthetist and I am grateful that in those excruciatingly painful-yet-precious moments with my daughter, someone was there to hold my hand. Someone wanted to know her name even though she wasn't breathing or crying.

So many before me have walked this road and, sadly, many will follow. But, my hope is that they can experience the gentleness and kindness of those two amazing ladies, similarly, as I did.

Comfort Beside the Pain

Annelise Boge

Acknowledge and appreciate all moments the family has with baby.

As I sit down to write the story of losing of our son and daughter, a feeling of being blessed washes over me, despite all the pain. I have been blessed by so many positive experiences with professionals, family, and friends over the past couple years as we've coped with losing Andrew and Annika. My friends have stepped up in ways that fill my heart and soul with love and strength and I've been connected with medical professionals who truly care how I'm doing and offer their support.

Andrew was my first pregnancy and we were so excited to become parents; I could picture myself as the mother of a little boy. However, from 16–23 weeks, I began having increased abdominal pain, until I was ultimately rushed to the hospital. Due to undiagnosed Crohn's disease that led to a perforated small intestine, I had an emergency bowel resection. Our son was born a day later at 24 weeks and 1 day, weighing 1 lb. 10 oz. Because of his many medical complications, we let him go the next morning. He passed in my arms and I was surprised by how substantial he felt despite his tiny size.

After much healing and many medical appointments, we conceived Annika, our rainbow baby, our second chance. My pregnancy went smoothly until 23 weeks, when she was diagnosed with duodenal atresia. It was supposed to be correctable by surgery following her birth. We even met with the same surgeon who had done my surgery. However, as my amniotic fluid levels continued to rise, I went into preterm labor at 28 weeks. Labor was thankfully controlled and I remained on bed rest in the hospital, continuing to have contractions and gradually dilate.

Annika and I bonded intensely during my nearly seven weeks of bed rest and we were surrounded by so much love and support from family, friends, and professionals. Suddenly, however, our world fell apart again when Annika didn't have a heart beat on morning monitoring at 35 weeks due to a cord accident. This was despite kicking just a couple hours prior. We were shocked and devastated and so angry to have lost a second baby.

Through all of the loss and trauma we've experienced the past couple years, the memories that repeatedly come back to me are of the professionals who celebrated my children and helped me to find the sweet and normal aspects of my deliveries.

The general surgery floor nurse, Andrea, chatted with us about choosing our son's name after his sudden, scary arrival and after whom we named our Andrew.

The NICU nurse who confirmed we'd done the right thing letting Andrew go after one day of life.

The labor and delivery nurse, Marlena, who called Annika by name while I waited for her arrival on bed rest. She, too, knew of Annika's sweet and mischievous personality traits, learned solely through her movements and habits.

My OB, who told me our daughter had lots of dark hair as she was crowning and confirmed she was so beautiful as she was born.

Nurse Robyn, who assisted during delivery, and captured such heartbreakingly sweet photos of Annika.

Alex, another nurse, who handed me a lifeline in the form of a Post-it note with her personal phone number on it the morning after Annika's delivery.

The scrub tech, Kendra, who has become a close friend. She assisted with my delivery of Annika and has been a source of hope and understanding

These professionals will always be intertwined with my memories of my children's births. Although there is tremendous pain and sadness involved with these deliveries, there are also many moments of sweetness and love. These professionals helped to make that possible. As we remember our son and daughter and struggle to build our family, it's these experiences that allow us to feel like parents, albeit not in the way we'd like. They provide us with some positive memories on which to reflect, and give us some small degree of comfort that our children were cared for and are still so loved.

Create Healing

Lauren Lane

You are the memory makers. Help create healing experiences.

Dear Nurse,

I know it feels like you've worked a million hours this week already; or maybe not enough hours, or you're spread across three different locations and have a board full of patients. You've had some fantastic ups and downs in the labor and delivery unit for sure, and you love your work, but that doesn't mean it's not really, really hard sometimes.

And why would it be hard when you're helping bring new life into the world? Surely isn't that full of joy? Apart from demanding patients, irrational expectations about delivery, or difficult situations out of your control, sometimes, on the rough days, there are patients like me — the moms who come in to discover devastating news. The days when the baby will come, but new life doesn't come with it.

Those days, they rock the patient's world, but I know they rock your world, too. No matter how many times you've been through it, it never gets easier. In fact, it may get harder every time it happens. Every time you stand in the room to assist a mom who is about to meet their much-awaited child with anticipation, but will eventually be met with tremendous grief. Incomprehensible grief. The kind that school couldn't train enough to help assist and the one situation in which you have no words to console them.

Nobody does.

You, even on the days when you've worked 16 hours straight, you still look right at me and tell me how beautiful my baby is, even if there is obvious evidence of her passing. You arrange for someone to come take pictures, a service I didn't even know existed. You help quietly shuffle the visitors around, somehow seeming to know when I need people in the room for support and when I clearly don't. You tell me you don't know why this happened, but you stop my mother-in-law from asking me and you deflect those answers to yourself, instead.

You go to the bathroom and cry, mortified that I might see you. Please let me see you cry. It's ok. It's good. It shows me that this precious little girl impacted others. Your tears show me how real and raw this is, and that my cascading emotions aren't out of the norm.

Here's what I specifically want you to know.

In my case, I was delivering a stillborn daughter. I'm about to be forced to make an entire lifetime of memories in one single day. Potentially two, if I'm lucky, and the hospital has the resources to allow me more time with my child. I got seven hours. I spend more time in an average day at work than I got for my child's entire life earth side. Please make it clear to me or to my support people how short this window is, because none of us are prepared for how short or how fast it is before that time is over. You can't comprehend that in the fog of trauma, shock, and grief.

I want you to know that I may seem out of it, but I'm attempting to commit every single thing to memory. That means this may be your average work shift, but for me, it's a day I'll replay in my memory until my own death. What you do and say today around my family and me, I will carry it for life.

I trust in you to be the good portions of those memories, or at least in the memories that don't make everything worse. Trust me when I say that while today is already hard, you have the power to make today tremendously meaningful or devastatingly traumatic. I trust that you'll help me and my family to make our time sacred, because that will either have the power to help me transform this trauma into healing or be something that keeps me stuck. Please don't even suggest that I could have done something different, that I or anyone else is to blame, or that I should do something when I'm not ready.

Don't force me to say goodbye if I'm not ready yet. Don't force me to talk about funerals or cremation when I'm just wrapping my head around labor. And please, just go slow. The slower you can go, the better. The faster you go, the less my foggy brain can catch up to what is going on. Love has a big part in helping me today, but tough love does not.

I am grateful for the moments you spend with my family guiding us through this loss that is bigger than life. You, dear nurse, are the connection between my family and our daughter. Please understand we need you to do your best when we are at our worst. Thank you for showing up and for knowing that while we do not get to leave the hospital with a baby in our arms, our baby is as important as the one that is in the next room crying. Because of you, the moments and memories you helped to create will be something that we forever cherish.

Thank you.

I Want You to Know

Alexa Bigwarfe

Be informed. Educate the family. Prepare them for all outcomes.

I think about that time often. I think about you often. The nurses who took care of me each day, who kept me company, surprised me on my birthday with decorations and singing and treats. I think about the doctors who rounded on me each morning. The med students who woke me up to take my blood pressure and to ask me the same questions day after day after day. I especially remember the techs who changed my sheets, made me feel fresh, and chatted with me when I was dying of boredom. And who could ever forget the sweet volunteer, an older woman from Germany, who came in on Sundays with magazines, ice cream, and sometimes even gave me a leg massage. I always felt cared for during that long and difficult stay, at least physically.

I also think a lot about the fact that even after spending almost five weeks on 24/7 monitoring of my baby girls, I was not prepared for one of them to die. Yes, I noticed that you all stopped talking about her future. I noticed that after the echocardiogram, not only did the doctor never come back to talk to me or tell me the results, but that the plans shifted from her going to a different hospital after birth for surgery, to no plans at all. I noticed. And I wondered why there was zero courtesy to fill me in on what was happening and why plans were changed.

In hindsight, while I am so thankful for the care and treatment you gave me, I feel there is one area in which you really dropped the ball. I don't blame you for this; I blame the lack of education and training. I blame our society's inability to handle death and grief. I blame ignorance. Regardless of the reason behind it, no one prepared me for what was to come. And, sadly, there are many gentle ways you could have been a part of helping me prepare for the inevitable.

It's important for me to share with you why I was in the hospital in the first place so that you can be best prepared when caring for families like mine in the future. Our daughters were monochorionic-diamniotic (MoDi) twins — one placenta, two sacs. They were diagnosed with twin-to-twin transfusion syndrome (TTTS) at 20 weeks' gestation. I found that many of my caregivers, if they had heard of TTTS, didn't really understand it. TTTS occurs in roughly 15-20% of MoDi twins, and, sadly, is the cause of more deaths of babies each year than SIDS.

The biggest problem with TTTS is that the babies do not receive an even share of the placenta and the fluids needed for survival. One baby is a donor baby, the other a recipient. The recipient receives excess fluids and this overload can cause heart failure and hydrops, which is what our baby Kathryn developed. Many donor twins also are unable to thrive and die from not receiving enough fluids.

TTTS is 100% fatal if not treated. There are multiple treatment options, including amnio reduction to try to level the fluids and a laser surgery to sever some of the shared veins. My doctor incorrectly assumed that I was ineligible for the laser surgery, and we were treated numerous times with amnio reduction instead.

There are so many complications that can occur with TTTS, from organ failure to hydrops, preterm delivery, and more.

I wasn't aware of these facts until much later, until after returning home without one of my babies. While our outcome can never be changed, I could have been much better prepared for Kathryn's demise, and certainly more prepared for what I could do to honor her after her death. It's my hope that sharing this information will help caregivers to talk to and share information with future mothers who have received a life-threatening diagnosis.

So, I want you to know a few things that will maybe make a big difference for someone else. These tips come from a place of love. If you're reading this book, you've already shown a commitment to wanting to understand and show compassion for the parents who lose their babies. And I thank you for that. These are simply suggestions based on my own experience.

Now I know you're not counselors or psychologists, but the fact is, YOU are the people who spend the most time with the mothers. And I could be completely off-base here, but I think that you should be prepared to give information to a mother who is perhaps not capable of bringing herself to even think about anything but having a healthy baby.

With that in mind, here are some things I want you to know, from the patient's perspective.

It's okay to help prepare a mother for the death of her baby. In fact, it should be something you have been trained on, so that if the moment ever happens that you have a mom on hospital bedrest and the prognosis is poor, you know what resources to tap, what steps to take. I understand that it may be scary, awkward, and downright uncomfortable to tell a mother that she should prepare for the death of her child. I understand that you may get negative feedback from some women. Some mothers may not want to talk about it at all. Tell them anyway.

I should have been better prepared for my baby's death. I refused to think about it. No, it's not that I refused, it's that I could not. And a mother shouldn't have to.

There are a few things that I wish the labor and delivery staff would have told me. I wish someone had taken the time to say, "Your baby is very sick. Our doctors are going to do everything they can for a positive outcome, but here are some resources to help you prepare for her death."

There have been some well-documented cases in the last few years of parents who were aware their baby would only survive a short time after birth, if at all, and chose to do some special end-of-life activities with their baby. You can direct moms and dads to look up those situations, or tell them about what happened and how the parents handled their short time with their babies.

I wish I'd known that I could have professional pictures taken with her. I want more than anything to be able to show a beautiful picture of my sweet baby in my arms, and I have nothing like that.

Nor did I know that there's no rush for the baby to be taken away. She could have stayed with me longer. We only had moments together. Moments. We should have had a lifetime, and we had moments. There was no reason for her to be taken so soon from my arms.

Do you know what I was doing for four hours of the precious few that my baby was alive? Trying to pee.

Yes, trying to pee. After four hours, I finally got a catheter and was relieved.

There are a growing number of resources available now to help parents navigate this horrendous experience. Perhaps you can request that they be purchased for the staff, so you have the resources at your fingertips. I don't know if I would have read a book like that or not at the time, but I do know if my sweet nurses spoke to me about the high possibility of my daughter passing, and took the time to discuss it with me, I would have thought more about the topic.

Despite the opportunities that were missed, I will never forget the kindness and love shown to me by my caregivers for those long weeks in the hospital. I hope that my advice to you will help you care even better for mothers facing horrible outcomes.

Firsts

Jessica Meyers

Celebrate every milestone with parents.

Firsts. They're something every new parent gets excited about. First giggle, first time rolling over, and first bath, just to name a few. When your baby is born 16 weeks preterm, those joyous "firsts" are replaced with a different type of firsts. Like first time off an oscillating ventilator, first time trying a nasal cannula, and first time outside the incubator. They're firsts that are also met with great fear, and without the cute picture with a catchy caption to post on social media.

Our daughter Paisley was born at 24 weeks while my husband and I were living abroad in Germany. We didn't speak much of the language, further adding to the stress and fear that having a child in the hospital brings. We struggled with being able to communicate our needs and to understand what was being said about Paisley's constantly changing condition. This was especially difficult with the nurses. After all, they are the ones who spent the most time with our child. So, losing the ability to properly communicate meant a lot was lost in translation.

One nurse, Sonja, holds a very special place in our hearts. She would attempt to tell us stories of things Paisley did during the night, stories she knew would put a smile on our faces and lift our spirits, but, once again, we were faced with the language barrier. So, she started taking pictures and printing them out for us as a way to help bridge the language gap. It was a small and simple gesture, one that didn't require translation because a picture can speak every language.

One of the photos Sonja gave to us was of Paisley without any CPAP or nasal cannula on. For the first time, she was breathing without any assistance, a moment I wish we could have been a part of. Because of Sonja, we were in a way. She was documenting firsts for us. In those moments, all my worries would melt away, making room for the joy and happiness that is felt when your child accomplishes something for the first time. What Sonja was doing for us was priceless.

During the course of Paisley's four-month journey, she gifted us with many firsts — like Paisley's first time wearing clothes. I would constantly ask the doctors when we could dress her. I would leave a bag full of cute little outfits, just in case. Sonja got the green light and surprised us with a fully dressed Paisley when we arrived. Every shift she would have fun getting her all dressed up for us. I soon found myself excited instead of nervous to walk into the NICU every morning. I looked forward to seeing what outfit Sonja had adorned Paisley with.

Sonja was on shift the night Paisley unexpectedly passed. She quickly ushered my husband and me into the hallway as the doctors attempted to save Paisley's life. All we could hear were the haunting sounds of a failing heart and doctors frantically shouting in a foreign tongue. I didn't want to believe what was happening. For the first time, I was so thankful for the language barrier I hated so much. As things grew calmer and quieter, Sonja stepped into view. With tears streaming down her face, she shook her head, confirming every parent's worst fear. The moments after we entered Paisley's room are foggy, but I will always remember looking up and seeing her with her hands over her face just crying. Paisley wasn't just loved by us, Sonja loved her, too.

When it came time to say our goodbyes, Sonja asked me to pick out one last outfit for Paisley to wear. I chose a soft pink nightgown, embroidered with a small pair of silver ballet slippers on the front. We didn't stay to see her dressed in it, in those moments my heart couldn't handle seeing Paisley in that way. It was a choice I soon came to regret. The next morning came and we went back to the hospital to take home her belongings, along with a card from the nurses. It wasn't until a few days had passed that I finally opened the card. Inside was Sonja's last gift to us. It was three pictures of Paisley sleeping peacefully in the pink gown I had laid out for her. The photos also captured Paisley's last first. The first and only time we'd ever see her face free of all tubes, and tape. Even in death, she managed to take my breath away; she was so beautiful. Because of these photos, I no longer have to wonder what was hiding behind all those stickers and tubes.

I will forever be grateful for the time Sonja spent on making sure our language barrier didn't rob us of the time we had with Paisley. I'm thankful for the things she did that made parenting Paisley from the NICU a little less painful. The pictures and memories of Paisley's firsts will always remain my most prized possessions.

Overwhelming Love

Marie Emmel-Frazer

Tend to parents, as well as baby.

My beautiful son, Cody, although he weighed only one pound, eight ounces, had an amazingly strong spirit. He was born premature, but the doctors said he was healthy and only needed care in the NICU to feed and to grow. My little man sat under the lights, with his knit hat and mask on. When I touched his soft skin and caressed his head, he felt like an angel.

I knew every night that I left the hospital he was in good hands, as his lead nurse, Nancy, had fallen in love with him instantly. She would leave us notes about his night and small treats for when we were there. We felt secure that our son was loved and cared for in our absence.

After a few weeks in the NICU, we got a dreadful phone call that something was wrong and Cody needed to be transferred. The doctors said he had NEC, which is an infection in the bowel. They had started him on meds, but he needed to be at a higher-level facility.

At the new hospital, we were offered a room to have 24-hour access to our son. My husband and I sat bedside and watched him grow to get better, only to then grow weak.

We prayed that he would have the strength for just one more day.

We prayed that the medicine that the doctors gave him would help.

We prayed that the blood he received would give him strength.

We prayed for him not to hurt anymore.

We prayed that we would be strong for him.

We prayed for us to be sick in exchange for Cody to be healthy.

The staff flocked to see Cody's golden glow. There was something special about him, but none of them could explain it. He held people's hearts in his hands and made them feel a sense of peace. He had a strength that we have never seen before or since. Cody had an incredible ability to calm one's soul by just being near him.

The nurses were not only our son's caregivers, but ended up being ours, as well. We spent hours talking, becoming informed, and being cared for by the nurses and social workers. They reminded us to take care of ourselves. They made sure we went outside for fresh air and would even ask us to lunch or to join them for a walk. At the same time, Cody's original hospital team would call to talk with us and to hear daily updates. I didn't feel like we were patients, but a family of sorts. We were extremely bonded to them.

As time progressed, a series of events led us to the most horrible news. The tears in the doctor's eyes, how he choked back his emotions, told us of the battle ahead for Cody. The doctors said that if he could survive 24-48 hours, they would attempt an implant surgery, but that it most likely would only help him survive a few short years. As a result, Cody could have liver and kidney failure and major medical problems during his short life, if he survived. He would be IV fed, and most likely never speak, crawl, or walk.

Our son looked so weak and pale. But, even though the doctors said he wouldn't respond to us, he opened his eyes! We tried not to celebrate, but all of us were hopeful. We sat with Cody and talked and sang to him. Friends, family, my husband, and I sat vigil by his bed. Our nurses put up separators and allowed all our visitors into the NICU. Nurses coming and going checked on us to make sure we were doing okay. Our social worker cancelled her evening plans to stay with us and even called the cafeteria to make food so we were taken care of and fed.

After a while, it was clear that Cody was losing his courageous fight and was only being kept alive by machines. He was bleeding internally and slowly dying. The nurses allowed my husband's grandmother to perform a sacred Indian ritual and for church leaders to give him a blessing. Our nurses asked if we wanted the staff to give them privacy. We wanted them to stay and spend time with us.

My husband and I talked to the doctors and nurses at length about how to ease Cody's pain and help with comfort so that he would not hurt any more. They spoke to us with honesty, open hearts, and love. After an informed conversation, we asked our families to say their goodbyes so my husband and I could be alone with him.

My husband and I took turns holding our son. He told Cody how much he loved and cherished him. I told him that it was okay to let go. He was so weak and frail. I sang him songs and told him how much I loved him and what fun new adventures he was now able to go on.

It was important to us that he died in my arms, singing lullabies to him, knowing how much his dad and I loved him. With tears in my eyes, I asked the doctors and nurses to remove his life support. As I watched the nurse remove the breathing tube from his mouth, I saw the tears stream down her cheeks and her try to control her breathing so that she could stay calm. The room was full of people, yet I heard no voices or monitor sounds. I saw people, but I did not see their faces. It was as if Mike, Cody, and I were all alone in a crowded room, in our own quiet universe.

Cody didn't even fight for a breath; he died in less than 40 seconds. It was the hardest thing to do in my life, but I knew I couldn't put my needs and wants for him to be here over his needs of having comfort. He was my little warrior.

Although we only had 52 days to hold his hand and to kiss on him, those were the best 52 days we have ever had. The love and support of the doctors and nurses allowed us to spend so much time with Cody and learn how special he is. Cody taught my family and friends so much. He affected so many people. He is an amazing little soul.

When funeral arrangements were finalized, we informed both

hospitals, even though we had been told that staff don't attend those events. To our surprise, almost every doctor and nurse that cared for Cody attended his service! Having them there meant the world to us and confirmed that they indeed held Cody with high regard. My husband and I continue to honor both hospitals on the anniversary of Cody's death to say thank you for the amazing support that we were given at such a difficult time of our lives. Without them, we could not have survived. We are eternally grateful for each one of Cody's caregivers for tending to our family.

Being Present in Letting Go

Trina McCartney

Create a sacred space for the family.

There are moments throughout our lives that contribute to the patchwork of our hearts, both the good and the bad. Then there are the moments that define who we are and that which we are made of. Some have the ability to take hold of us, chew us up, and spit us out in the lonely, dark wilderness leaving us feeling numb, shocked, disoriented, lost. Some even leave us struggling to breathe. The year 2013 had many of those moments for our family.

At a routine 30-week ultrasound, our baby was diagnosed with a massive intracranial hemorrhage from a then-unknown brain tumor. I was left in the room, alone, trying to absorb all that was just said, waiting for my husband to arrive. Our world went from a planned home-birth with a midwife, to that of ultrasounds, MRIs, blood work, fetal echoes, a team of medical specialists, consultation upon consultation, tears upon tears, and disbelief upon disbelief. I knew this could happen, but not to us. Not to our baby. Not to our family. Our youngest daughter's diagnosis was worse than we could imagine: severe disabilities, semi-paralysis, hospitals, specialists, and rehabilitation. We were asked if we knew anyone with special needs. No, we didn't. We felt alone. How quickly dreams full of excitement, bliss, and anticipation transformed into uncertainty, confusion, and so much fear.

Weeks passed and we moved through and into our new reality. We read. We asked questions. We researched. We prayed. We were introduced to an amazing team of medical professionals, including an invaluable nurse practitioner, who became our main point of contact as we navigated the medical system pre-birth. She was our lifeline during this time because of her empathetic, compassionate demeanor. Ironically, she was once a midwife, so she was a perfect fit for us. We became hopeful. We prepared ourselves for what everyone called the "new normal."

Our beautiful tiny being of uncertainty was born on May 23. What was for certain, however, was that we loved her with abandon. We named her Katelyn, meaning "pure one." She was born via C-section and surprised us all. She needed no immediate medical intervention. She was utterly perfect. It was as if the doctors had misdiagnosed her. We had four days of this amazing bliss of uncertainty. We were so incredibly hopeful.

Unfortunately, the doctors were not wrong. The days that followed were both more awful and more wonderful than I could have ever imagined. Those moments played together in chorus. They were full of medical procedures and surgeries. Scans, X-rays, NPO, tubes, lines, boluses, transfusions — words I wish I didn't need to know. Sleepless nights and endless tears. Fear and helplessness. But they were also full of light and love: holding our sweet baby, visits from our older children, caring notes, meals, music in the hospital healing garden, a nurse's shoulder to cry on.

We were given a family room in the hospital. We will be eternally grateful for this space to rest, to escape, to breathe. It became our temporary home. We journeyed alongside Katelyn's nurses and doctors. They became an extension of our family. They loved her. They loved our family. They treated her with such tenderness, and us with such compassion and kindness. We became very close with one nurse named Erin. Erin often knew what we needed without us even having to ask. After a day of strict instruction not to touch, talk, or move our daughter, Erin made it possible for me to hold her, in the middle of the night, despite her extreme fragile state and countless tubes. Our breathing synchronized, our heartbeats became one. I am not sure if

Erin will ever know how special this moment was to me and how it is forever etched into my heart. She made the impossible, possible. It was at this moment that I knew, if we had to, she would be the one we would eventually hand our baby over to.

After two days of what seemed like a downhill battle, we decided that there would be no more medical intervention, only touches of love for our baby girl. Since we could not leave the hospital, Katelyn's nurses set up a beautiful private space to spend her last hours. There was a full bed where we could hold and snuggle her, soft music, starry night-lights, and enough space for those close to us to attend a special blessing and to say their goodbyes. We asked Erin if she would be there, not yet realizing the extent of comfort that her gentle presence would provide and how we would replay that night, and her loving involvement in it, over and over in our minds for years to come. This sacred evening became pivotal in our healing journey.

On May 31, our brave daughter ended her battle and took her last breaths in our arms surrounded by her siblings, extended family, close friends, and her nurses. Our hearts shattered for the loss of possibility, the dreams, and the physical touch of her tiny body that we would never feel again. Her last moments, although incredibly heartbreaking, were also so peaceful and beautiful. It was a night filled with so much love. Erin said that it was tangible, as if you could feel it move throughout the room. Together, with Erin, we made foot/hand casts, fingerprints, bathed her, and took photos with our baby. I am eternally grateful for those eight days we had with our Katelyn and the space that we were gifted to spend our time together.

We are still in touch with Erin. She has since taken a position in bereavement for perinatal loss. In her latest email to us: "Katelyn has provided me with this very special opportunity to work with families who are struggling with losing their own beautiful babies. I feel so lucky. So, I need to say thank you again to you for including me in your life and to your beautiful baby for having imprinted herself on my heart." No, Erin, it is us who feel so lucky. You are a gift to those experiencing the unimaginable.

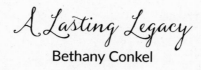

A Lasting Legacy

Bethany Conkel

Be familiar with neonatal organ donation. Have resources available to inform parents of their options.

Although our story is unique in many ways, the actual situation surrounding our story really isn't all that different from ones you as a care provider have encountered in your career.

It starts with a young pregnant couple … Over-the-moon excited. Joy oozing from every pore. They are going to have a baby!

But, sadly, an early ultrasound reveals a fatal fetal anomaly (in our case anencephaly). During the ultrasound, the parents are clueless and are still exuding joy and excitement.

Unfortunately, you as the medical provider have to deliver the gut-wrenching news that no new parents want to hear — news that will turn their world upside down.

Their baby is going to die.

You offer your condolences … and their options: termination, compassionate induction, continuing the pregnancy. You tell them to think about it for a while. You may or may not show your bias on which option the family should choose. You feel badly, there's nothing you can do to change the outcome, and, honestly, it comes with the territory. Not every baby lives.

Although for the medical providers this was a sad-yet-familiar situation, for us, it was life-changing news.

That evening, we sat with our family, utterly devastated. Bewildered. Sideswiped. Lost in a fog of emotion. Not sure of how to move forward.

This was our first baby. The first baby for all three sets of grandparents and the first niece or nephew to our siblings. This was not how things were supposed to turn out.

Our world was upside down.

That same evening, my phone rang; it was my OB. He called to check on us. This meant so much to me and made me feel supported and cared for, especially since we had only met him for the first time that day.

Despite the diagnosis, my husband and I made the decision to carry our baby to term. But not JUST carry to term, we decided we wanted to be the best parents we could be and love our baby as much as possible. We wanted to make enough memories during the pregnancy with our baby to last an entire lifetime. To do this, we made a "bucket list" of things to accomplish before our baby was born. We would go to the zoo, camping, swimming, hiking, kayaking, attend a monster truck show, see a concert, play on a playground, putt-putt golf, eat special foods, and go to favorite restaurants. We would read books, do things that involved the grandparents, the aunts and uncles, and our close friends so they could all make memories as well. We even had a 24-week "Life Day Party" in lieu of future birthday parties, complete with a huge cake and all the decorations. For us, this allowed us to have joy during a time that is typically filled with sorrow.

We wrote monthly update letters to keep family and friends informed. Each month we sent a copy to our OB's office to make sure they were included in our journey. Often, our OB, the nurse, or the secretary would comment about something we said in our letter or ask if we had any special plans coming up. It made us feel like they really cared about our pregnancy and us.

Not only did we want to make the most of our baby's life, but we also wanted to make the most of our baby's death. So, we decided to pursue neonatal organ donation and whole body donation. As you read this, you might be shaking your head and saying to yourself "that's not really possible." And you aren't alone — that's what we were told by many different care providers. Not one of the providers we spoke with could give us solid answers, so we did lots of research and made tons of phone calls, but to no avail. Finally, after several months of searching, a genetic specialist got us connected with our local organ procurement organization (OPO).

Sadly, our OPO told us options were limited. They said that the only option would be a tissue donation (heart for valves) if a six-pound weight requirement were met. We knew this was unlikely, as our baby was measuring in the first percentile in most growth categories. Despite this, we still felt very strongly about donation. We asked about donation for research in the form of a whole-body donation. Again, we were told it wasn't possible. We asked if there were any options. Our OPO looked, but was unable to find anything for us.

As the pregnancy came to an end, we held a palliative care meeting with our OBs and a team of other providers from our hospital. Everyone wanted to make sure our desires were met, and that everyone knew the plan in advance. We went over my lengthy birth plan and asked a ton of questions. They were so patient with us and tried to show care and empathy. This meeting helped us immensely. But, it still did not help us with our final desire of organ donation.

Then, three short days before my scheduled C-section, I decided to pick up the phone and make one last phone call to an organization my OPO had briefly mentioned. It was a Hail Mary, last-ditch effort phone call … and it became the call that changed everything.

That call opened the doors for our baby to donate liver, pancreas, and whole body — each to a different researcher! We were ecstatic. We had felt so strongly about allowing our baby to have an impact on the medical community, and that desire had finally come true. It was the icing on the cake! Our OPO was so gracious and took care of all the details at the hospital to make this option viable.

The day to meet our baby arrived. The two leading OBs in our practice performed the C-section together. They wanted it to go as quickly as possible to allow for us have as much time as we could with our baby. After delivering our baby, they placed our son on my chest and let me hold my boy during the rest of the procedure. It was love at first sight.

Our son lived about 80 minutes. He was surrounded by love for every second of those minutes.

After he passed, my husband had the privilege of walking him to his recovery surgery and handing him to the recovery surgeon. After the recovery surgery was over, our baby boy was brought back to us for more bonding time. We spent the day celebrating. We took pictures, got hand and foot prints, and even had a full birthday party complete with cupcakes, a birthday boy hat, and 24 people crammed in our tiny room to sing happy birthday to our sweet boy.

At the end of the day, we said our final goodbyes and allowed our boy to go on what I call his "internship", also known as whole body donation. He was gone for eight months before we received his ashes back.

Over the past several years, we have had the amazing privilege to learn a little about his donations. His whole body donation allowed for a new location for a pediatric life-saving procedure to be passed through the FDA. His liver went to study cirrhosis and liver disease. His pancreas helped with discoveries regarding type 1 diabetes. His donation ended up being a catalyst for a new neonatal research donation program to open up! In the four years following his donation, more than 75 other families across the United States have been able to let their babies donate organs and tissue to research because of that program.

We named our son Amalya Nathaniel Conkel — Amalya is Hebrew for "work of the Lord" and Nathaniel is "given by God". In our eyes, he was truly a "work of the Lord, given by God". Although we know our son's life always had inherent and intrinsic value, for us, donation added an extra layer of meaning to his amazing 37 weeks in utero and 80 minutes in our arms. He now lives on through his donation.

As I said in the beginning, our situation was fairly common from a medical perspective, but our story ended up being very unique. The outcome of our story happened because we received support from our care providers both in our OB office, and at the OPO. Although they did not always have the answers to our questions, they always supported us. They created an environment that made us feel like we could pursue our wishes for our baby, our pregnancy, and our son's legacy. My hope is that other care providers will continue to provide similar support.

Above & Beyond

Tricia Winkelman

Support the family from start to finish. You become part of their story, part of their child's family.

Let me tell you about Nurse Taylor, a NICU nurse at our local hospital. I can't think of a more gentle and kind soul. You see, when we met Taylor, our daughter Emaleya was on life support. We were so scared, like in a bad dream. Our daughter was connected to tubes and IVs and we were afraid we'd hurt her if we moved or held her. All I wanted was to hold and comfort my three-day-old baby girl. She needed me.

Taylor was right there to comfort and guide us. She helped us time and again with the transfer from the small hospital bed to our arms. She was happy to do so every time. She talked us through diaper changes and sponge baths, always staying close just for reassurance. She held my hand through all of it. Taking the time to just sit with us and gently remind us that we needed to get rest and eat. Reminding us so that our bodies were rested and minds were clear. We knew that if we left that room that Emaleya was in loving hands.

It was found that our daughter had a rare genetic disorder and nothing could be done to save our sweet baby. And when we were given the news, Taylor was there at our sides, once again. To this day, I'm not sure if nurses are usually asked to join the group of doctors when they give this news to families, but there she sat, like the doctors, trying to maintain composure as the devastating news was delivered. She was a rock for us and she became an honorary auntie to Emaleya.

When we made the decision to remove our angel from life support, we hoped Taylor would be with us. It was her scheduled day off, but she made it clear, she'd be there no matter what. She saw that all of our needs and wishes were met. When the moment came, and my daughter had left this world, Taylor drew a bath and we washed and got her dressed. We sat for a while, Taylor, too. We knew what would happen next; someone would need to take her to another part of the hospital for the organ donation procedure. I couldn't watch them take her. So, I placed my beautiful baby girl in the arms of my sister. She stayed in the room for a while longer just holding my daughter, her niece, unable to let go. Taylor stayed, too. There stayed the two aunties comforting each other to say their final goodbye. My sister told me how all the other doctors and nurses had stopped in to also say goodbye to my angel and many did it with tears in their eyes. And then the moment came for the staff to have to take her. Taylor promised my sister that she would take her personally, as my sister didn't want her to go with strangers. Taylor kept that promise.

I look back and realize that this was a difficult day for her, too. I think she had only been on the job a year. She had not gone through this yet. You would have never known it though. My family will never forget her kindness and compassion. In fact, we're friends to this day.

As I was leaving the hospital that night, I handed her a pair of Emaleya's shoes. I don't know what possessed me to do it. But, a few weeks later, I received the best text from her, a picture of her Christmas tree, with the most heartwarming ornament, Emaleya's shoes. Our daughter left a footprint on Taylor's heart, too.

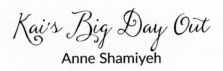

Kai's Big Day Out

Anne Shamiyeh

Create memorable experiences for the family. Make the impossible, possible.

"So what you're saying is, you do not see life for our son beyond the walls of this hospital?" The answer came quickly and with great certainty, "No." Tears flooded my eyes and my heart raced. It was difficult to breathe. My husband respectfully looked around the room and asked if we could please have some time alone. All of the bodies cleared the room.

Just four and a half months after coming into the world, we learned that our son, Kai, would not be coming home with us. We felt angry, shocked, and defeated. It was beyond what our minds could comprehend. We didn't know how long Kai would be with us, but we did know that we had to make the most out of every day that he had left.

One of our first meetings after that day was with palliative care. The only experience my husband and I had had with palliative care in the past was with our own parents. My husband and I had both lost a parent to cancer over the last decade, so going into this meeting, I felt very shut off to the team's input. It made the end feel too near. After four and a half months of fighting for his life, it felt as though we were giving up on our son. That made me feel anxious, like we didn't believe in him, or recognize his strength. But what it truly meant was that we were making it okay for him to let go.

They asked us to make a wish list of things that we wanted for Kai. I couldn't think of what we might put on this list until they started giving us ideas, like give him a real bath, immersed in water, or taking him outside. What? Outside? Kai had a trach and was permanently attached to a ventilator and, as far as I knew, kids with vents didn't get to go outside. He had more tubes than I could count and I just hadn't realized that any of these things were possibilities. Until this moment, we had only been told what Kai couldn't do and, suddenly, doors were opening that we didn't know existed. Normal activities that we take for granted with ourselves or our other children seemed like Christmas for our fragile boy.

Weeks of preparation went into planning "Kai's Big Day Out." We were warned of all the possible things that could go wrong and even had to sign a DNR. There were so many moving parts to this event that had to be just right to make it happen. We pretty much had to be ready any day, any moment. The event required two nurses, a doctor, a respiratory therapist, myself, my husband, Kai's nana, two sisters, a photographer (and good friend), and a portable ventilator. It was quite a production. Not your everyday walk in the park.

There was a small courtyard on the sixth floor of the hospital and it was the only outdoor spot still within the hospital. Chances were it would be gloomy there, as the hospital is situated in one of the foggiest parts of the city, but that day, the sun shone like I hadn't seen it in weeks. We spent exactly one hour outside, where we held Kai on a bench, put a tiny pair of sunglasses on his face to shield the sun and we laughed. A lot. It was the most normal day we ever had as a family of five. Time stood still. It will forever remain the most cherished day of my life.

The palliative care team gave our family hope for Kai. Not an unrealistic hope that he would one day come home with us, but the hope that we could make the end of his life as normal as possible. Nothing is normal about spending your life in the NICU for almost six months and never getting to go home with your family, but to allow us the comforts of bathing our child in a baby bath or spending time with him outside — those were things we had only dreamed about doing with Kai. The love and care that our nurses and the palliative care team showed to our family will forever make the hardest days of our life the most beautiful. No amount of thanks will ever be enough.

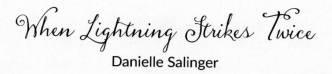

When Lightning Strikes Twice

Danielle Salinger

Be present. Take time to explain and prepare family for what to expect.
Respect this sacred time.

"I'm here for you. I'm not going anywhere."

My memory of the many moments while in the hospital are vague; too little sleep and too much adrenaline, heartbreak and fear. They blend the memories together like a painting by Monet, giving only the vague impressions. But I remember the words that our nurse, Anna, said to me as she sat in the chair beside my bed and took my hand.

"You're my only patient right now. We can wait until you're ready."

Her words struck me most because they were in such stark contrast to how things were handled two years ago, when we found ourselves in quite literally the same position. At that time, things happened so quickly it was hard to understand, to come to grips, to accept, to breathe. I was 21 weeks and 3 days pregnant with our son, Josiah. We were so excited to be having a boy after three and a half years of trying to get pregnant, following the harrowing birth of our daughter six years prior — a birth I nearly didn't survive due to severe hemorrhaging and a cervical tear.

We were so concerned with my own survival through another birth that we never thought about the possibility of something happening to our son after we crossed that first trimester threshold. Then my water broke in the middle of the night. We rushed to the hospital and were taken immediately to labor and delivery. I was examined and, once the situation was explained to us, we were given options. I could stay in the hospital on bed rest, hoping to hold onto Josiah until he had a better chance of surviving, we could give birth to him and have an opportunity to say goodbye, or we could terminate the pregnancy. Those choices dwindled in less than an hour when I began to heavily bleed. After the trauma of my first birth, the doctor became concerned about hemorrhaging.

We were told that the best way to ensure the chance of my own survival, since there was no hope of saving our son, was to terminate the pregnancy immediately. There wasn't time to ask questions, or consult our regular doctor. We were terrified and devastated, and made the decision we thought would be best for our family, although we didn't fully understand the choice we were making. The doctors and nurses and staff grieved with us. They were caring and kind, and took wonderful care of me as I was prepped for surgery. However, the prep was only for surgery, and not for the shattered pieces of me that would remain.

Looking back, I could see that the care was only for me, and not my son. He was not viewed as a patient, or even as a person. The only tangible evidence I had that he existed were the ultrasound photos and the prints of his hands and feet that a nurse was thoughtful enough to make sure we had before we left. That wrecked me, because I needed to grieve a person that wasn't even truly recognized by those that were helping me. A little over six hours after we had arrived at the hospital, we were discharged home and I left empty and ill-equipped to handle the way that my life had been cleaved apart.

They say that lightning doesn't strike twice, but in tragedy, this isn't true. This is how we found ourselves back in labor and delivery, two years later, facing the loss of another son. I was 19 weeks and 4 days pregnant on the day Lincoln died. While so many things were different, it was all very much the same. We would still be leaving the hospital without our son. This time, it was my cervix that gave out, instead of the amniotic sac. I had arrived at the hospital the previous day, and we tried all night to save him. By the next morning, it was obvious that there was nothing else that could be done and I was going to give birth that day.

"What's going to happen now?" I asked Anna. As she turned in her seat to face me, she clasped my hand between hers.

"Whatever you need," she replied. "Would you like to meet with a social worker?"

"Yes, please."

We never met with anyone other than nurses and doctors when Josiah died, but this time we were able to speak with a professional who guided other families through moments like these. Sitting in our dark room, we discussed resources and support. We reviewed mortuaries and end of life tasks that are often forgotten. We talked about counseling and bereavement groups. We were given these tools in order to reach out to our community and find the resources we needed to survive well. We were also given a folder with the same information, since we certainly wouldn't remember later. But she knew we would need it eventually, and we did.

"Would you like to meet with a minister or priest?" Anna asked.

"Yes, please."

We lost Josiah without any spiritual guidance, but Lincoln was blessed before he was born, which was of great comfort to me. The minister came to our room and sat beside me to talk about our son and our losses. We shared with him the circumstances of how we lost Josiah, and the wracking guilt of choosing to terminate a fiercely wanted pregnancy. We also discussed the too-soon-to-be loss of our son, Lincoln, and our fears for what would come after; fears of having to tell our daughter, and other family and friends, that we had once again lost a son, as well as fears of navigating the compounded grief we were facing. He listened and he commiserated. He offered guidance, thoughts, and a bit of faith for what was to come; faith that we needed, but had been missing for some time.

"Would you like something for the pain? I know you're hurting right now, but there's no need for you to suffer physically," Anna assured me.

"Yes, please."

Once the epidural was in place, I told her we were ready to meet Lincoln. We didn't want to prolong the inevitable, and wanted to allow him to go peacefully as we held him.

"How is this going to go?" I asked.

She could have glossed over what we were about to experience. She could have used terms we didn't understand. Instead, she was blunt and she was thorough. And she prepared us as best she could, both physically and emotionally, for what was about to occur.

"Would you like me to bathe him?" she asked. "I could also place one of the gowns we have on him."

"Yes, please."

She honored Lincoln. Not only did Anna honor us, our family, our experience, our past, our birth … she honored our son. She saw him, and she saw us, she saw our love, and she made sure to mirror that back to us. She knew that we were going to leave the hospital in pieces and knew we would have to be put back together. Through every step, as slowly as we needed to go, she made sure that some of those pieces would be imprinted with Lincoln, to carry with us always. She gave us memories of love, thoughts of future healing, and a small piece of her to carry with us as well. She taught us that when lightning strikes twice, it's time and care that can make all the difference.

When Joy & Sorrow Intertwine

Nichole Davis

Reduce future regrets. Guide families to spend quality time with their baby.

My husband Tim and I had been married for five years and after a three-year struggle with infertility, we were blessed with our son, Colson. When we decided to start trying for our second child, we were beyond thrilled that it happened so quickly. At my second ultrasound, there were two strong beating hearts! We could not believe it — twins!

At around 18 weeks, we found out we were having identical girls. We learned the risks associated with identical twins and were assigned a high-risk specialist, but everything was going smoothly. We chose their names, Callie AnnaMarie and Coley Louise, started their nursery, and had baby showers. I could tell who was who when they moved and kicked. Callie was head down on my right side and moved constantly. Coley was breech on my left side and was the calm one.

One evening, I started having close, intense contractions. Tim rushed me to the hospital. The nurse found both girls' fast strong heartbeats and that my cervix was closed. At 31 weeks and 5 days, there was no need for him to take the girls. The longer they stayed inside, the better. I was sent home with medicine to stop the contractions and told that if they started again to call him. I had some contractions the following day, but nothing major.

Two day later, when the contractions were closer and more intense, we headed back to the hospital. A nurse hooked me up to the monitors and found Callie's heartbeat right away. She had a tough time locating Coley's, but kept trying. Finally, she found it and gave me a warm-hearted grin. I relaxed a little, but when another nurse came in, she realized it was my heartbeat instead of Coley's that the previous nurse had picked up.

While she was searching, our doctor walked in and the nurse updated him on our situation. He started examining my belly. After a couple of minutes, he called for the ultrasound technician to bring in a more enhanced machine. At that point, I started to feel more concerned, so I called my mom and informed her of what was transpiring. The technician scanned and scanned for what seemed like an eternity, keeping a poker face the whole time. Our doctor then stated, "I'm so sorry, her heart has stopped beating!" Those soul-destroying words have forever altered our lives. I stared up at Tim, hoping he would tell me she was just fine, but with tears coursing down his cheeks, I could see it was undeniable.

I felt like I was not in my body at this moment, like I was observing someone else's tragedy, not ours. Our little girl, dead? Impossible! She was safe and sound two days ago! I have never encountered an emotion that could come close to describing that moment in time. When my mother arrived and I uttered the devastating news, I don't think it registered until she held our deceased daughter after the C-section.

Callie was born first, full of life. Coley was born silent only one minute later. Only glancing at her for a brief minute, Callie was handed off to the NICU team. Tim held Coley while they stitched me up. He cradled his lifeless daughter, looking at me with the emptiest expression I have ever witnessed upon his face. We were moved to the recovery room, where our doctor personally carried Coley to us. She was donned in the most angelic gown I had ever seen, hand sewn, with the fabric of a wedding dress.

We spent time alone with Coley before our family came to say hello and goodbye to our daughter. Anyone that wanted to hold her did, and the hospital took pictures for us. My time with her was so concise that still today, all I want to do is hold her again, admire her beauty, and tell her how much I love her. She was so perfect.

Losing a child is deeply heartbreaking and confusing, as well as physically and emotionally exhausting. I remember most of our four-day hospital stay, but some remains a blur. We were overwhelmed by the countless difficult decisions we had to be make.

Did we want an autopsy?

Did we want the hospital to dispose of her remains?

Did we want to have a funeral?

What outfit did we want her buried in?

What funeral home did we want to use?

What did we want her obituary to say?

We had just lost our daughter, while our other baby was in the NICU fighting for her life! How were we expected to process all of this at one time? Our brains were completely shut down and we were just going through the motions.

The hospital's motto is to serve with compassion and that night was no exception. We received the best care by the entire staff during our stay. Although they did not lack in compassion, they sadly fell short on how to facilitate a bereaved family. The hardest part of my grief journey, aside from missing Coley, is the regret I have from our hospital stay. Because I did not know to ask and the staff did not know to educate me, I missed out on making my final memories with my daughter.

I never got to change Coley's diaper, bathe her; put clothes on her, read her a book, rock her, put a bow in her hair, sing to her, take a family photo, take a photo of us holding both babies, or just hold her for as long as we could. The only pictures we have of Coley are the ones the hospital took for us, for which we are grateful. They also gave us every item that Coley came into contact with: her blanket, brush, booties, the donated gown, a hair clipping, measuring tape, etc. But, no one ever asked us if we wanted to make final memories or even told us we had those options. I wish someone would have come to talk to us and told us to think about the final memories we wanted to make, because I now regret not making these for the rest of my life.

Callie stayed in the NICU for 15 days and when it came time to bring her home, it was bittersweet. We were so joyful to have our miracle baby, but we felt full of sorrow that we weren't bringing her sister home with us, too. I have a physical reminder every time I look at Callie; we are missing her identical twin. I fight a battle between joy and sorrow every day.

I never want a family to regret the things I do, so my husband and I helped implement a Butterfly Nursery in memory of Coley at the hospital. The Butterfly Nursery is a room designated for families whose baby has died; it looks more like a nursery and less like a hospital room. The room is furnished with a full-size bed, TV, rocker, child's table for siblings, baby bed, bookshelf, and a Cuddle Cot™. It is supplied with books, hand and foot molds, bath tub, bath essentials, journals, diapers, wipes, ink for making hand and foot prints, bows, and bowties. A brochure given to families includes our story, along with resources and recommendations for memory making. We have transformed the room into a peaceful, loving place for families to spend time together.

My desire is that other hospitals will learn of this room, recognize its importance, and provide a similar space to their patients. The way bereaved families are cared for will impact their entire grief journey and the day they lose their baby will forever be imprinted in their mind. They will experience enough just by losing their child. It's important to be comforted. The medical community is viewed as being strong, but it's important to show emotions. Do not be apprehensive to show emotion when you are with these families. It will indicate that you truly care.

I view life through a different lens now and analyze things differently. My whole life is eternally changed because of the traumatic journey I continue to wade through. Some people may think I am a strong person, but I am strong because of the continued support system that stands beside us and encourages us to continue to keep moving forward. Without them, this road would be much, much, tougher. Coley is on my mind and in my heart, all the time. Although I am delighted to have two precious, healthy children here on Earth, I constantly struggle with not having Coley here, too. I will forever feel blessed that God chose me to witness the beauty of having two very special girls grow inside me.

Ten Sacred Hours

Sharon Cox

Photographs are irreplaceable. They are treasured beyond measure.

There are moments in life that irrevocably change the way we look at the world around us. Losing my beautiful son Ethan to stillbirth forever changed me. He was so wanted, so loved, and already such a part of our family. I never imagined that with just a few words from a doctor, our world would forever be changed.

On the day Ethan was born, I felt such a contradiction of emotions. It was one of the darkest days felt in the deepest part of my soul. Nevertheless, it came to be one of the most precious of days. I was finally able to see my son, hold him in my arms, and fall deeply in love with his sweet face. Ten hours to memorize everything I could about him. Ten sacred hours.

There are so many things that I remember about that day. The doctor's tears as he broke the news that there was no heartbeat. The gentle, tender way the hospital staff interacted with us. The card on our hospital door; a leaf with a teardrop to communicate with others that we had lost our baby. Those around us offered so much love and comfort.

I will forever be grateful to the nurse who recommended that someone in the family go home and gather something personal that we could dress or wrap Ethan in when he was born. She encouraged us to bring a camera to capture pictures of our son. I knew immediately how important this would be for all of us. We had walked into the hospital completely unprepared, thinking that it would just be a quick check-up. No bags, no clothes, no camera. Her encouragement, in that moment, was such a gift to our family. While I was in the early stages of labor, my husband made a quick trip home. He made it back soon, and it was a comfort to know I would be able to photograph my boy when he arrived. We didn't know what to expect, or what Ethan's delivery would bring, but we couldn't wait to meet him, even though his birth was surrounded by such heartbreak.

Holding my son in my arms for the first time broke my heart wide open. There was a deep realization that this day of his birth would be the only one I would get to spend with him. I never wanted to forget the way his little hand looked, curled in mine. I wanted to memorize every single curve of his face and the color of his hair. I had been so afraid that I would forget the details. I was so thankful that I could photograph my beautiful boy; yet, even at that time, I didn't truly understand how meaningful those pictures would be to our family.

Those photographs, captured in the most tender of moments, spoke volumes. No words could express the emotions and pure love reflected in the pictures of my husband holding his son for the first time. The beauty and wonder reflected in the sweet photograph of my two-year old daughter reading a book to her little brother is something words couldn't have described. The sorrow expressed in the photograph of the great-grandparents holding our boy, with tears streaming down their faces, tells their story most eloquently. These pictures show what words could not express in that moment. I photographed Ethan's little toes, his long fingers, and his beautiful face. I captured the way his left ear curled sweetly, and the little swirl of his hair. He looked just like his daddy, but in little form. Those photos tell a story. Our story. They are sacred. They are love.

Today, if you come to our home, those photos are hanging on the walls. They are tangible expressions of how deeply we love our son, and how much we miss him. He is not forgotten. They open opportunities for us to share about how intensely his short life impacted us. For the dear family and friends that could not be there to meet him in person, these pictures bring comfort and a connection to our son. They are gentle, warm reminders that we have and love three children. In that brief, ten-hour span of saying hello and goodbye to our boy, those pictures are one of the few things that we can hold in our hands.

I know so many people would have the thought, "Why would I want to capture one of the most heartbreaking days of my life? Why would I want to remember all that pain?" When I look at those pictures, pain isn't the thing that stands out strongest. It's pure love. There may be tears, heartbreak, and grief in the background ... but there is strength, beauty, belonging, and truth in clearest focus.

They say a picture is worth a thousand words ... a thousand words? Grieving parents will tell you a picture is worth so much more. I couldn't have possibly understood how much having a photograph of my son would mean to me in the days and years to come. For my family, a picture is worth ten sacred hours.

Your Name Matters

Rosie O'Brien

Say baby's name. Write baby's name. Refer to mom and dad as baby's parents.

Ariana. My firstborn. I love saying your name, the way it looks written down, and the way it's spelled ... the way it sounds. Ariana; it is beautiful, like you.

It was the morning of Valentine's Day, 2014, when we found out you were coming. We had waited patiently, and to our surprise, the time had finally come. We were going to be parents. We were finally going to start the life we had always dreamed of. I was in complete bliss. The love I felt for you was instant and new. In one instant, my love for you transformed the world and everything made sense. This chapter of our lives was the most memorable, innocent, and pure. I am eternally grateful to have had such a wonderful pregnancy with you. Your dad and I spent those months dreaming of a life with you, doing all the "last things before baby" and preparing for your arrival. We took all the baby classes that were offered at our hospital and spent those evenings walking, sharing, and being excited for your arrival. Every day, we were a little bit closer to holding you, rocking you, finally seeing you in that little blue dress that was so thoughtfully picked out for you. We built a castle for you. These were the words from your daddy.

Our time visiting the hospital was made even more special knowing your abuelita would be there to help deliver you. My mama, Rocio, worked in the labor and delivery department, so we felt like royalty. It was a feeling, but even more than that really. The best way I could describe it is like ... an extended family. We loved visiting labor and delivery, and getting to hear the sounds of newborn babies. I couldn't wait to hear your cries. All the nurses greeted us with the biggest smiles and shared in their friend's excitement. You see, my mom had only been waiting forever to be an abuelita; I could almost say she was more excited than I was. Almost.

"Hi, my name is Sandy, I will be taking over now. Is it okay if I update your board?" I rolled onto my side, slightly aware of the time. I had been asleep for what felt like hours, but I still felt the effects of the drugs. As I looked up, I saw Sandy. Her hair was pulled back and she gazed down on me with gentle eyes. She had just started her shift, although she looked tired. The lights were dim, but I could see that her eyes were red and I wondered if she had seen my mom out in the hall. I wondered if she had held her and cried with her. My mom had always told me what a close-knit group of nurses she had the pleasure of working with. Angels, they are all brave angels. Sandy repeated the question. "Is it okay if I update your board?" After a moment, I realized what Sandy was asking. "Sure," I replied. "May I write the names of everyone present in this room?" she asked. "Yes. Rosie. My name is Rosie. This is my sister Janet, and my dad, Jean-Paul," I said. "And what is your baby's name?" she asked. Suddenly, I was flooded with emotion. Sadness, devastation, confusion, and maybe even a little anger filled my heart. I was overwhelmed. My throat closed up and it was difficult to breathe, but I managed to respond.

As soon as I said "Ariana", I burst into tears, the first real, hard tears I had shed after being in shock. After hearing the doctor tell me the day before, "I'm sorry. There's no heartbeat." I turned back over and buried myself in my sister's arms and just cried. Hard. I felt everything. In that moment, I questioned whether my heart would be able to endure this pain. How could I survive this? How could I leave this hospital without my baby? Without Ariana.

I was so distraught that I was kept medicated to calm down. We had made the decision to go ahead with induction and when my contractions first began, I thought Ariana was kicking. "I can feel her! My baby is okay!" I shouted. Then I realized, no. Those are contractions. It was the first time I felt what I thought was a kick in two days. The contractions I felt were not her little legs kicking anymore and they were growing in intensity. I was devastated. I had to prepare myself for giving birth to Ariana. After all, I had waited for this day for 40 weeks and five days. We had waited for this day for years. Looking back, even though that particular moment crushed me, I appreciate that Sandy asked and was respectful enough to add Ariana's name on the chart that only read "fetal demise."

Fetal demise. It was not what I expected to see on my board. But, of course, what expecting mother to an otherwise healthy baby ever does? I wasn't sure what to think when it first appeared on the board. And when Sandy asked me, I was a little angry and maybe even questioned her sensitivity to what we were going through. But, of course she was sensitive. She did something for me that, at the time, I didn't know I needed. I needed to know that she validated my baby, my Ariana. As a loss mom, that is one thing I keep going back to. Her name. Her name matters. It is important to hear. It is important to know other people recognize that she existed, and that her memory still exists. So, I'm thankful for Sandy, for knowing what I needed, and for honoring my Ariana.

Handing Her Over

Amie Lands

Parenting continues beyond life.

"Can I have the honor of holding your baby?" the nurse asked, as I handed my daughter over for the very last time. I watched myself from outside my body as I handed over my most precious girl while the world slipped from under my feet.

Isabella was an amazing nurse and she gave the biggest hugs, the kind that envelop your whole body and you wish would hold you forever. The day my daughter left us, Isabella's shift ended at 3 p.m., but she knew what we felt aware of; today was the last day with our daughter alive. So, when 4 p.m. rolled around for our daughter's next round of meds, Isabella was waiting for the call that our daughter had died.

She entered so respectfully, explained what to expect in the moments after death, and asked if I wanted to bathe my baby girl one last time. I was scared, but also knew I wasn't ready to say goodbye, so I followed her lead as the expert, since, obviously, she was.

An aroma of spearmint and lemongrass radiated from the bath. The softly tinted water was warm to the touch. My daughter's body gently rested as Isabella placed her in the tiny tub. She demonstrated the sacred act of bathing my daughter, the last ritual I would perform as her mama while she was earth side. It was breathtaking and my honor to bathe my daughter's perfect body. It was also devastating.

I dressed my sweet girl in her last diaper and most beautiful gown, the one that she was supposed to wear home. Instead, I held my daughter with her weight heavy upon my chest for hours as I stared out the window watching the sun fade and the moon appear to light the night.

And finally, reluctantly, the time had come. My husband and I were exhausted. After 33 days of limited sleep and heightened anxiety, we decided it was time to say goodbye.

That walk down the hall, I knew what was coming and I wanted to stop time. My broken heart was just beginning to feel the magnitude of what was to come. Isabella's words were the only reason I could stomach handing over my daughter. It was "her honor" to hold my sweet girl.

And then I proceeded to vomit.

Isabella was only one of the many incredible nurses to care for us during the time with our daughter. Her commitment so greatly, positively impacted us during what can only be defined as the most beautifully heartbreaking time of our life. Because of the support we received, we are surviving. We have survived the unsurvivable.

Nurses are human, too. I can only imagine how any of the staff felt when they left work that night to return to their families. I will never forget how I felt that night. Despite the devastation, the heartbreak, and the most tremendous pain I have ever experienced, I also felt loved. I felt Isabella's love for my daughter and for my family. Isabella's words will forever be remembered. It was her honor to hold my beloved child.

Holding is Healing

Stephanie Tower

Give parents important information in every way possible. They will need to reference this in the future. Encourage time to say goodbye. These moments cannot be returned.

Our second son was conceived right on schedule. We plan everything, so why wouldn't he be perfectly timed, too? His pregnancy also blessed me with a gigantic kidney stone, which I was going to have to wait until after he was born to have removed. This meant I had intermittent excruciating kidney pain throughout my pregnancy. He arrived about 4 weeks early (not in the schedule); however, he was healthy as a horse and such a beautiful little ginger. We named him Oliver, calling him Ollie from the start.

At his two-month checkup, Ollie received his vaccinations on schedule and I spoke with our beloved pediatrician about how well he was doing. He was a much better sleeper than our first son and he also ate more efficiently, so my breasts saw little pain this go around. I probably knew what I was doing, as I'd had practice with my first son, but either way, Ollie was such an easy baby. I told my pediatrician that I sometimes let him sleep on his tummy, as he was already so strong, pushing up on his arms and lifting his head already. Our pediatrician wasn't concerned about his tummy sleeping, due to his health and strength.

When Oliver was ten weeks old, I had the kidney procedure to remove the stone that plagued me during my pregnancy. I pumped and dumped the milk following my procedure, as I had been under anesthesia and my nurse said it wasn't safe to give Ollie. I was on pain medication the days following the procedure, but labor and delivery stated that that milk was fine to give him. I worried about Ollie being exposed to the medication, but breast milk is liquid gold, so I pumped away after I was released from the hospital.

It was a Friday and I was home recovering from the procedure the day before. The kids were at daycare and my husband was at work. I got a call from the police saying that Ollie had been transported to the hospital from daycare and I needed to come right away.

When my husband and I arrived at the hospital and the chaplain walked in the room, I knew Ollie wasn't alive. A chaplain doesn't come to tell you how your child is doing; they are there to tell you they're already dead. I was also certain it was my fault, as I had given my daycare provider the pumped milk from when I'd been on the pain medication. I worried about giving it to him, but since it had been cleared by the hospital nurse, I sent the milk with him. The doctor said that it's too early to tell, but Ollie's death appeared to be SIDS-related. I knew better, though, and felt I'd never be able to forgive myself.

When the hospital staff came in to ask if we wanted to hold Ollie to say goodbye, I didn't know what to do. I just sat there and stared blankly at my husband and my friend. The detective's partner, a woman, leaned towards me to say, "I wouldn't if I were you. You won't want to remember him that way." I wasn't sure what to do and was frozen in fear and shock. I decided not to, as the woman suggested, but my husband wanted to hold him. He went with my brother to say goodbye, while I cried with my friend. It was one of the worst decisions I've ever made.

My heart ached to see Ollie, my breasts throbbed with milk to feed him, and my arms longed to hold him. I buried my face in his blanket so I could gather his smell, which was all that was left of him.

At the funeral home, a few days later, the director said that Oliver's body was there. I felt hope.

"Can I hold him?" I asked.

He said no and that it was against the law, he couldn't allow it.

I could think of nothing else but getting to hold my baby one last time. Knowing he was in the building and not being able to hold him was too much to bear. My friend explained how I hadn't said goodbye to him, and if they could please make an exception, it would mean so much to me. After some discussion, he understood.

My husband and I were led into a room, and they seated me in a rocking chair. The director said I must stay in the chair and warned me Ollie would look different, as he'd had an autopsy and a knit cap would cover his head, which had been examined. He also said that he would be cold, as this is how they store the body. Moments later he brought me Ollie, bundled up in a blanket with a cap on. He was placed in my arms and he was so cold. I got to stare at his beautiful sleeping face for the last time. I rocked him with my husband standing next to me, memorizing his every feature one last time.

I wish I had taken that moment when he was warm and looked more like himself at the hospital. I would give anything to go back in time and take that opportunity when it was offered. This moment of closure helped me to understand that he was really gone, giving me just one last moment with him. My arms stopped aching to hold him. My heart will never be the same, but my arms stopped longing.

The days that followed Ollie's death was an absolute blur and haze. I was in and out of the ER multiple times a day with complications from the kidney procedure and my house was flooded with loving supportive people. It was determined that Ollie died from SIDS (which in and of itself is saying the doctors didn't know why he died), but I knew that it was my fault for giving him my pumped milk.

In one of my many ER trips, my people surrounded me. These were the people that were keeping me alive, as I didn't really have much will to live at that point. Our pediatrician came into my ER room. In all honesty, I don't remember what exactly he said to me, I was on so much pain medication from my kidney issues and utterly numb from the loss of Ollie. My amazing friend had the idea to record him, so I could listen to what he said later and really be able to hear it. What I do remember, is that he sat down with tears in his eyes and literature in his hand to say, "I heard you've been blaming yourself for Ollie's death and I'm here tell you and to show you that it isn't your fault."

No one was going to convince me Ollie's death wasn't my fault. I still wonder sometimes if I had done this or that if he would still be alive. I didn't feel an actual release from pain until the autopsy came back saying that there was zero pain medication in his system when he died.

It meant so much to me that our pediatrician took the time to print off the research and come to speak with me directly, caring so much for my heart that he wanted to help ease my pain.

In the most devastating of moments, parents are looking to the professionals to guide them. Please guide them to healing with less regret. I want all professionals who ask a family to decide whether or not to see their child's dead body to know how important this is. It is the opportunity for a parent to say a final goodbye. I am forever grateful to the funeral director who bent the rules and gave me this opportunity. I can't fully explain in words how crucial this moment was for my acceptance that Ollie was gone and for my overall healing.

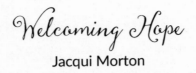

Welcoming Hope

Jacqui Morton

Be prepared with referrals and resources for when the family returns home.

It was Jeanne that told me to care for myself as I would have cared for the baby I couldn't hold. Her name was on the half-sheet of paper given to me by the midwife's office at the follow-up appointment, which I scheduled because it felt like someone should check on me after the procedure, though no one was asking to.

I was in shock. My body was, as in had been, pregnant, growing what I was sure would be my daughter. My belly was hard and round, though still small — and then it wasn't. Soft. Empty. Sitting in a waiting room full of big blooming bellies. Unsure how to be a mother to my two-year-old boy; trying to just move forward, but somehow feeling a piece of me had gone missing, or been taken — leaving me unable to mother.

I hated myself for feeling so stuck. I'd only been just over 15 weeks pregnant. I was angry with myself for being so angry. It had been so early. I, like those around me, thought I should just move on.

I'll never forget Jeanne's cheerful voice. When she returned my call, she asked if I was experiencing postpartum depression. She explained she only sees women of reproductive age, and is often referred for this reason. I stood in my kitchen as I searched for the words to explain myself.

It was my second pregnancy. My first baby, my son, is now two. He was hard to conceive. This pregnancy happened quickly, almost by surprise. But something felt off from the start. The first prenatal appointment and ultrasound were fine. The midwife suggested scheduling the early ultrasound and quad testing to screen for chromosomal abnormalities because I was going to be 35. At the ultrasound, the doctor was concerned. We had the CVS testing that day. I was contracting. There were so many things wrong with the fetus. We learned she had Trisomy 18. We didn't want her to suffer. We didn't want our son to lose his baby sister. We decided that to be her parents, we had to let her go.

Although she had been physically removed from my body, Jeanne helped me understand, I hadn't truly let go of her. Perhaps some piece of me was frozen, never processing beyond the diagnosis. I knew all the words and facts that I had read. The images of the babies who survived were carved in my mind. The picture from the genetic counselor's office, the third copy of the chromosome that changed our family, would be with me forever.

But I had become dissociated from my body, where she had lived. For just over 15 weeks. Once I heard she'd likely not make it, or might die soon after birth, or would perhaps not have a first birthday, or ever live independently, I had gone numb. It was too difficult to live through, so only some part of me had.

Jeanne helped me visit my loss experience just closely enough to remember and somehow hold the darkest parts, though I could barely speak them: The protesters that we passed as we drove into the hospital that rainy Thursday morning. The very pregnant administrator who conducted the intake interview — her question about how we would prevent future pregnancy was my first clue that no one in the clinic seemed to know that mine was not a wanted abortion. The waiting for my cervix to ripen. The doctor who appeared to confuse me with another patient. The not knowing what happened to her remains. The sadness that friends and family didn't know what to say or do.

The not asking. The guilt of not asking. The questions.

Why didn't I ask about footprints?

Why didn't I ask what would happen?

Why didn't the doctor seem to understand?

Why did it feel like I was suffocating in a secret?

Just to say them out loud helped me feel better. It had happened. Her life passed through mine. Just like that, in 15 weeks. Jeanne asked if I wanted to name her. I did not. At that time, I felt that I could not — that the only way to name a baby is to meet the baby. In choosing to say goodbye early, I had given that up.

Jeanne helped me realize how angry I was that I wasn't given more choices about my choice. Why didn't I ask about waiting until I could be induced — to meet her, name her, and say goodbye? It's the ultimate question. And then what? This is the question that always follows. Jeanne helped me see that there was no going back. There was only forward. I could both honor my loss and my sadness, and move forward, with self-forgiveness. In her office, I vowed to write about my experience, to find meaningful ways to honor this little spirit that I hold so close, and to love my sons as well as I am able.

I got pregnant again, quickly, perhaps on purpose because of my age, or perhaps by mistake because the hole left in my soul was so large. I saw Jeanne and walked my way through that pregnancy. She helped me find hope for another healthy baby and when the anxiety of being pregnant again was almost too much for me to bear, Jeanne helped me return to my breath.

Jeanne and I talked about how we often must go to the darkest places of our sadness to reach the light. When I brought my second son to meet her, it seemed I had come full circle, and I eventually let go of my visits with her. Recently, I received a letter that Jeanne was retiring from her practice. I felt a sense of sadness, for the things I haven't gotten to tell her about, and a deep sense of gratitude, for her wisdom.

Aching Arms & Broken Hearts

Gail Whetstine

Offer a weighted item. Give empty arms something tangible to hold.

How does one even begin to describe emptiness — not only of heart, but also of one's arms? The utter cruelty and grief that accompany being wheeled out of the hospital without your newborn baby — twice — defies description. The passage of time is irrelevant when memories — both of heart and body — come flooding back with even the mere mention of pregnancy or infant loss. Experiencing two pregnancies ending in loss due to prematurity, acquainted me all too well with aching arms and broken-heart syndrome.

My ever-so-brief moments with my tiny infants (which were, literally, minutes) can be likened to a butterfly that lands on you. Upon noticing its presence, in the blink of an eye, it is whisked away by a gentle breeze, leaving you almost breathless and full of wonder as to where it is off to next. Almost as soon as it comes into sight, it is gone, leaving you drenched in gratitude for its delicate beauty and for choosing you as a brief resting place.

My pregnancy losses left me with few concrete images but, rather, voluminous unfulfilled dreams. Although I had a sense that my babies were with me in the ethereal after-life, I lived with a sense that they were "out there," and obviously separate from me. Sometime after my losses, my encounter with The Comfort Cub®, a weighted teddy bear, immediately took me to a place in time when comfort was not to be found — anywhere. The moment the bear was placed in my arms, its weight and softness brought a sense of a tangible grounding that caught me totally by surprise.

This was not just any teddy bear. The Comfort Cub suddenly turned my long-remembered emptiness into a moment of earthly connection. There was a comfort and satisfaction upon embracing this bundle of cuddliness. Immediately, I was compelled to gently rock to and fro, as any mother does with a baby in her arms.

Nothing can ever replace the precious daughter and son that I lost, but holding the weight of The Comfort Cub has offered a path to healing and comfort for a long-held aching wound. Feeling its weight on my chest has had a restorative effect on my aching heart and empty arms. I am grateful for the gift of healing and comfort it has brought to my life.

Making Memories

Katie Ward

Create memorial items with the family.

Atop the changing table in Liam's room, a room to which he never came home, sits a beautiful decoupage box with a satin ribbon tied to hold it closed. Its contents hold my most treasured mementos of my son's life. Given to me on the day of his memorial service by our treasured team of nurses, are perfectly casted molds of Liam's precious hands and feet. They are so life-like; looking at them takes my breath away. Each line and wrinkle is visible, his little finger nails perfectly traceable. Every detail that I could hope to remember is there, replicated in these molds. They are the closest physical reminder that I have of what it was like to touch my son.

In the moments after my son passed, I remember being asked if I would like to have a mold of Liam's hands and feet. I said yes, but in my shock and despair, I declined to stay and make them myself. That is one of my biggest regrets and I feel angry with myself when I think about it. So, when the beautiful box was given to me at Liam's service by one of the most special nurses, I was overcome with gratitude. She said to me, I stayed with him for a long time. That thought and these molds have brought my heart tremendous comfort. Knowing that our nurses were so invested in our little family, I imagine it must have been difficult for them to take part in such a project. Yet, they set aside their emotions to create something for us that would create a tangible piece of Liam, an act of selflessness that gave us a completely priceless and irreplaceable gift.

I go into Liam's room often to look at his little hands and feet. Sometimes I stare at them, wishing that they were just a project done hastily with a wiggling baby instead of a perfectly still work of art created once my son's heart no longer beat. Other times, I close my eyes and trace over them, each detail committed to memory, reminding me of touching his feet when he was alive. I place my finger in the curl of his and remember what it was like to have those little fingers wrap around mine, a memory that makes me float away, smiling. Although I will always long for more, I will forever be grateful to the nurses that made these treasured mementos for us.

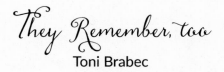

They Remember, too

Toni Brabec

Help families remember their babies. Create, participate, or refer families to local remembrance events.

It had been a long day. It had been a long journey. Yet, it was only just beginning. I looked down at my daughter, our little Olivia. She was perfect. Other than being born at 33 weeks and only three pounds, one would never know her kidneys were missing and her lungs had hardly developed.

I was roughly 20 weeks pregnant when we were told the news of Olivia's fatal condition. She was moving and kicking inside me at that moment. She was alive, and yet they were telling me our baby was going to die. I found it hard to believe at first. But she was feisty and lively. She was doing everything a growing baby should be. So how could she be dying?

Thirteen weeks later, she arrived. My husband and I knew the odds were against her, yet we held out hope that there might be something we could do. Despite all efforts, there wasn't much to do but to just love her and hold her until it was time for her to go. We didn't know how long she would be with us. We weren't even sure if Olivia would be born alive or still. But our baby was born and she was alive. I felt eager to meet her, yet dreaded it at the same time, because I would soon have to say goodbye.

Throughout my pregnancy and since we found out about her diagnosis, I naturally worried about a lot of things. I've never known anyone to experience anything close to this, so I felt like a deer in headlights. Stuck. Frozen. I was unsure of what to do or where to go. I had so many questions.

What if there's still a chance she could live?

What if she's born still?

What would she look like?

Would I get to hold her?

What would life be like after she was gone?

I worried that I would lose more than just her physical presence from this earth. I worried I would lose what emotional connection I had with her, that I would forget her or forget what it felt like to carry her, to be her mother. I was afraid if I lost that connection and those memories, then I would really lose her forever.

As we held her, whispered we loved her, she slipped away into eternity. She lived with us for nearly five hours. The time we spent with her was peaceful and full of love. The doctor confirmed her heart had stopped. Our baby was gone.

Lisa, one of the NICU staff, said she was going to take Olivia for a while, but that she would bring her back to us so we could spend as much time with her as we wanted. Reluctantly, I let her go. But knowing I would get to see her again made it a little more bearable.

I was brought up to my recovery room and was getting settled. Lisa came back up with Olivia and presented a box to me. I opened the box that had been decorated for Olivia. Inside were items we could keep; her name tags, little beanie hat, footprints, and a lock of hair. They had also made a mold cast of her feet. Items that we could take home and keep with us forever. That box, as simple as it may have seemed, carried a bit of my world of Olivia and gave us a way to remember my baby.

But it didn't just stop there. Lisa then handed us an invitation. She explained that the following week, the NICU department would be holding their annual remembrance event for all the families who had lost their baby while in NICU. Because we were so fresh and new to our grief, she understood that it was too soon for us to attend. But, Lisa offered to honor our baby in our absence by sharing a photo of our choice and reading a poem, scripture, or message for Olivia. I was blown away by how much they had already done for us and they were offering to do more. We took them up on their offer and submitted a photo and passage to read.

A week or so after, we received two videos from Lisa. The first video was of our NICU nurse, Jodine, reading the scripture passage and standing beside a projected photo of our Olivia on a screen. We could see in the video the number of families who came to attend and immediately sensed that this event was important to the families. The second video was of Jodine releasing a butterfly in honor of Olivia in a beautiful and peaceful setting among the other families. It was beautiful. We are so grateful that Lisa and Jodine would create and capture those moments for us when we couldn't be there ourselves. It meant so much that they cared enough to do this for us. My husband and I knew we needed to attend the next year.

We have attended every year since. And each time is so special to us. This is a time to meet other families who are also grieving, to sit amongst each other in solidarity. We come as strangers, yet we already know so much about one another. We get to see our babies and celebrate their lives, acknowledge their value to us. There are many activities planned for the families aside from the slide show and butterfly release: crafts for the siblings, keepsakes to take home, a scrapbook page made for each baby so family can write messages to their baby year after year, and a star chosen and named to honor our babies. The NICU staff knows how badly parents and family members need this. We need to come together to remember, honor and celebrate each precious life. They know we need to support one another and reconnect with each other and to reconnect with our birth workers and medical teams, and most of all, our babies.

As much as they invest so much time and energy to do all of this for us, what it has really shown me is not only do they care about us by creating an event to remember and honor our babies every year, but they also value our babies' lives just as much as we do. They remember them, too.

Caring Inspires Hope

Rachel Crawford

Honor each baby, their life, and their memory. Be compassionate, kind, caring, and honest.

One year after Aubrey and Ellie died, I attended a memorial for all the babies that passed away in the NICU of their hospital the prior year. I brought my son, Dustin, who was just three and a half, to honor his sisters — my sweet daughters — and reconnect with the doctors, nurses, and staff that were now woven into the fabric of my story by the saddest circumstances imaginable.

It was hard for me to accept an entire year had gone by. It felt both longer and shorter at the same time. It was a lifetime, really, yet seemingly in a blink, one year had passed. I sat listening to the speaker attempt to comfort the grieving parents in the room. He was the current head of the NICU and I could tell he was uncomfortable, although he spoke eloquently. He talked about how parents just want to know their babies are safe and nothing tips the world on its side more than the death of an infant. I can't remember how many babies he said died in the NICU that year. All I know is that two of them were mine.

I sent Dustin down the aisle to collect the gifts presented to honor the memory of each baby. We were the only ones there collecting two of everything; two balloons, two roses, and two wind chimes. I was so touched that the hospital honored Aubrey, too, as she was eventually transferred from there and had died in another hospital. Yet, they made sure she was included with her sister Ellie and didn't allow her to be forgotten on a technicality. Aubrey's hospital didn't have an annual memorial and I think it would have been a blow to my barely beating heart not to honor both of my babies that day.

When I just couldn't take it anymore, I scooped up my smiley little boy with a balloon in each hand and began the long walk back to the parking lot. It was one I knew well. The sound of our footsteps in the hall, the voices in the courtyard, the bench I used to sit on and cry with my social worker — all of it — was there to remind me. This time, everything reminded me not of their deaths, but of their lives, which felt like a wounding and a healing all at the same time. This was the air they breathed and the only home they ever knew. These were the people who know they existed, who called them by name, who stayed up all night looking after them, who stood in the hallway until I came out of that tiny room to hand over my little Ellie with tears and hugs waiting. They were Aubrey and Ellie's doctors and nurses, but to me, they were the proof that my girls didn't just die, they lived, too.

I wish I could say that all my interactions with doctors and staff were meaningful, but that would be a lie. The head of the NICU at Aubrey's hospital kept calling her "Audrey," no matter how many times I corrected him. He was stoic, jaded, and agitated during every interaction we had with him. After Aubrey's second brain hemorrhage, he sat us down to tell us what kind of life was in store for our little girl and it wasn't a good one. As we sat processing, we asked him what he would do if Aubrey was his daughter and he said, "Oh, you don't want a child like this. You are still young. You can have healthy babies." Even writing it now, hurts. I don't know if I was more angry, shocked, or sad, but probably all three, and the callousness of his words crushed the last ember of my dwindling hope. People can be so heartless. And heartlessness leaves scars.

After Ellie died the social worker assigned to me made plaster casts of her hands and feet. They are my most treasured possessions. Since Aubrey died at a different hospital, I was only given a lock of hair and smeary footprints on a tile. There isn't a day I don't wish I had plaster casts of her hands and feet as well. Aubrey's keepsakes felt like sloppy seconds, like obligatory hospital protocol, and it bothers me still. Ellie's keepsakes felt worthy of her. I don't understand why the quality of aftercare varied so widely between the hospitals.

Since Aubrey and Ellie died, I've served on a few panels helping hospital staff improve the emotional care of families with babies in the NICU. I say the same thing to the staff and doctors every time: Be a human first and a medical professional second. I think doctors and nurses feel so much pressure to fix problems, save lives, and even reframe tragedy, that they forget about the human experience in between. A baby should never be reduced to just a tiny patient. A terrified mother should not be treated nonchalantly. A frustrated father shouldn't be told to just calm down. A clinical approach simply isn't enough. We should always be striving to do better because hope isn't in technology and medicine, it's in hugs, caring glances, and incubators decorated with stickers, ribbons, and glitter glue by nurses not afraid to show me how much they love my girls.

It has been nine years since my girls died and in those nine years what has comforted me most is knowing that their lives mattered. Their lives were short but meaningful and I choose to live every day of my life better because they lived, not ruined because they died. The moment the doctor told me that my babies were coming early and we needed to do an emergency C-section to give them the best chance possible, life as I knew it was over. I was terrified. I gave consent and my sweet doctor shifted into gear. Truly, I've never seen such transparent focus and concern. He was serious but not stoic. As my heart sank I looked up and said to him, "This isn't good, is it?" And with tears in his eyes, he looked straight at me and said, "No honey, it's not." That moment of real human emotion didn't scare me like maybe it should have. It comforted me in an indescribable way. I knew I was in the hands of a feeling, caring doctor who was brave enough to not only tell me the truth about my circumstance but also show me the truth about his heart. His job wasn't an easy one, but he faced it with all he had in him. I committed to doing the same in that moment.

I have many regrets in the two weeks Aubrey and Ellie were alive, but the conversation with that doctor isn't one of them. He set the tone. His display of emotion gave me permission to display my own. His courage gave me courage. His honesty exchanged my fear with fortitude. His concern gave me hope. If only all medical professionals knew the power they have to set those they encounter on a path of emotional healing that surpasses any medicine or procedure they can provide. If only all humans knew that. You don't have to be a doctor to help. All you have to do is care. Caring inspires hope. And hope has made all the difference for me.

Part Two

STRATEGIES FOR HEALTH PROFESSIONALS

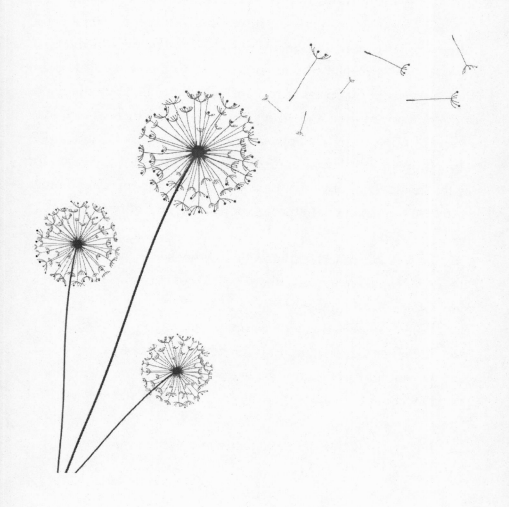

FOR EASE AND FLUIDITY, the choice has been made to refer to baby in the feminine. Doing so will help the flow of reading by maintaining a single gender throughout this part of the book. This choice was carefully considered and is not intended to exclude any precious baby boy. It will, however, maintain the consistency necessary to focus on the content of this section.

Infertility & Miscarriage

THE PREGNANCY JOURNEY BEGINS LONG BEFORE CONCEPTION.
ALLOW MOM TO BE AN ACTIVE PARTICIPANT IN HER CARE.

When a woman imagines the future possibility of having a child, it often seems so easy. But, many quickly learn this is not the case. When you see a patient in your practice or in the hospital, you are only seeing her at that particular point in her journey to motherhood, not the amount of time and struggle it took to get there. There may be years of hope, heartache, physical and emotional pain, and severe disappointment. It is important to have empathy and compassion for how far she has traveled, only to experience loss once or several times over. When interacting with those experiencing infertility:

- Be patient
- Review her chart before meeting with her
- Ask if she'd like to talk about past experiences
- Offer your condolences
- Deliver information with compassion
- Refer her to local support resources and/or groups
- Do not offer platitudes or assume that there is another chance
- Direct her to online support websites such as *Still Mothers* (www.stillmothers.com)
- Follow up with a phone call after initial care is received

ALL LOSSES, NO MATTER GESTATION OR AGE OF BABY, ARE WORTHY OF VALIDATION. VALIDATE ALL LOSSES.

When a woman becomes pregnant, she becomes a mother. She is carrying life inside her and chances are, she and her partner are planning for the future. Not only do they schedule birth classes, but many times they also plan or have a baby shower, collect items for baby, buy baby clothes, decorate a nursery, and visualize the life ahead of them. Their capacity to love has swelled and their vision for their future has been adjusted. It doesn't matter how long a woman is pregnant before she forms an attachment and connection with the embryo or fetus she is carrying; this is her baby.

Miscarriage is often an overlooked type of loss. When a pregnancy ends, innocence is shattered. The safety that she may have felt in the world, along with the belief that pregnancy equals baby, no longer exists. It is devastating and traumatizing and she needs acknowledgement that the grief resulting from this loss is real. For mom and dad — their baby has died, along with the hopes, plans, and expectations for the future of their family. This is a tremendous loss and whether it is her first or fifth pregnancy or first or fifth miscarriage, the grief that accompanies this pain is often dismissed.

It is also important to acknowledge that for some women, this pregnancy may have occurred after years of infertility or treatments, or a last effort to grow their family biologically. Acknowledge and validate her pain.

- Be patient during your visit
- Talk to mom
- Don't minimize or assume how she is feeling
- Ask her about her journey to become pregnant
- Acknowledge her loss
- Offer local and online support resources

- Include contact information for any remaining questions
- Follow up with a phone call

Sharing Devastating News

DISCOVERING A LIFE-LIMITING OR FATAL PRENATAL DIAGNOSIS
IS LIFE CHANGING. SUPPORT FAMILIES IN THEIR GRIEF.

The moment a family hears that their baby is not "perfect" is devastating. There are no words to encapsulate the loss parents feel when they learn that their baby will not survive, or if they survive, that their quality of life is questionable. Families instantly transfer from excitement to a crash course in medical jargon. For many parents, this means that they quickly have to learn about procedures they have never imagined and then are expected to make life-changing medical decisions that they were never prepared to make. And many times, these decisions are without guarantee that their child will survive.

The grief families experience happens immediately. As soon as the words leave the doctor's mouth, lives have been irreversibly altered and innocence is lost. Anticipatory grief begins as a family loses the life they thought they would have and fear sets in.

The waiting time that families endure is physically and emotionally taxing, not only for the parents but their extended family and any living children they may have. It is important to ensure that parents are tending to their basic needs during these chronically stressful times. Eating, hydrating and resting need to be encouraged so that families have the proper energy to sustain themselves. In order to be present and make fully informed decisions, parents must be of sound mind and being properly cared for physically will help them to do so.

Parents are asked to make impossible decisions when a fatal or life-limiting diagnosis is discovered. Regardless of the choice that a parent makes during this time, their immediate grief is as a result from anticipating the loss of their baby. Grief can often be compounded when parents feel forced to make medical decisions that they never imagined. Understand that every single moment, a family is potentially second guessing their decision and will need reassurance.

- Include entire medical team when relaying a life-limiting or fatal diagnosis
- Relay information as soon as possible, don't prolong the inevitable
- Suggest parents bring a third party to join them for support
- Advise parents to record conversation for later reference
- Give information verbally
- Have written explanations ready for parents
- Refer to fetus as their child
- If baby has been named, call baby by name
- Be clear, direct, kind, and loving when speaking about baby's prognosis
- Don't offer false hope
- Speak sensitively when offering pregnancy choices
- Don't assume parents will abort the pregnancy
- Don't assume parents will carry to term
- Offer resources that support families who end a wanted pregnancy
- Offer resources that support families who choose to carry to term
- Encourage time to discuss options. There is no rush unless medically necessary
- Give families space to deliberate
- Introduce the social worker to family to offer immediate support and resources
- Offer counseling to help with decision-making
- Support parents, regardless of their decision

- Empathize with the grief that parents are experiencing
- Offer contact information for additional questions
- Schedule a follow-up appointment with entire care team to ensure grief support

After the family has returned home without baby, an alternate reality sets in. It takes time to wade through the sea of shock and grief that they experienced while in the midst of their loss. Following up with the entire care team encourages parents to ask any remaining or new questions that may have surfaced as time has passed. It also allows them to see the impact their child had on each person who cared for their baby. It can reassure parents to know that their baby is valued and remembered.

INFORM PARENTS OF ALL OPTIONS. SUPPORT THEIR DECISION.

When the outcome is dire, asking parents to make a decision regarding their baby can feel impossible. Parents want to be assured that their child will be okay and when they have to look at statistics and odds to decide their child's fate, the decision becomes larger than life.

There is no such thing as too much information. Parents need to be informed of all options possible when considering potential outcomes — best and worst case scenarios.

- Encourage families to record the conversation to replay later
- Invite a third party to support the family when introducing information and options
- Be clear when explaining; use laymen's terms
- Draw pictures for clarity
- Give real life examples of every possible scenario
- Refer families to other parents who have made similar decisions, whether in person, online or through books

Parents are making life-changing choices and they will replay these conversations in their mind for the rest of their life. Do not hold back, this is no time to sugarcoat the truth.

When a decision is made, regardless of the outcome, support parents in their choice. Every parent makes their choice out of love for their child. Be sure to remind them of that when they doubt themselves — which will most likely be the rest of their life. Much of the support offered to those who end a wanted pregnancy, as well as those who carry to term, can be universal. Both choices end in loss and families each suffer grief as a result of that loss. Be sure to offer resources that aid in healing.

- Suggest that families document time with baby:
  ◦ Record baby's heartbeat
  ◦ Take maternity photos
  ◦ Make a belly cast
  ◦ Have a blessing ceremony
- Refer parents to bereavement counseling
- Prepare families for labor and delivery or ending a wanted pregnancy by using a modified birth plan. Consider using a birth and bereavement doula. Both of these resources can be found on the *Stillbirthday* website (www.stillbirthday.com)

Ending a Wanted Pregnancy: Families who choose to end a wanted pregnancy agonize over this heartbreaking decision. Their child was a much-loved and anticipated baby. Abortion is often decided either because of a poor maternal prognosis or to avoid the pain a baby may endure due to their diagnosis, should they be born living. Whether this decision is a medical necessity or made out of love for their child, it is an unwanted act.

Many times, moms who end a wanted pregnancy feel stigmatized and unworthy of the complicated grief that follows because abortion is not a universally or socially accepted practice. The trauma of aborting a wanted pregnancy is real and moms need emotional support. A tremendous amount of healing and normalcy can be found when connecting to others who have experienced a similar loss. Direct parents to find personal stories from reputable websites such as *Ending A Wanted Pregnancy* (www.endingawantedpregnancy.com) or *A Heartbreaking Choice* (www.aheartbreakingchoice.com) while simultaneously encouraging them to avoid the dark corners of the internet.

Carrying to Term: Families who choose to carry to term experience the daily reminder that the child they are in love with will die. Many moms find that memory making and honoring baby the remainder of the pregnancy can offer tremendous healing. It is also important to share the unique benefits of perinatal hospice and palliative care so that families have support the entire duration of mom's pregnancy, during baby's brief life, and in the time following their death.

While mom's partner may be able to compartmentalize the impending birth of their medically fragile baby because he/she is not pregnant, for mom, every encounter in public often includes unknowing passersby asking about her pregnancy. This daily interaction is exhausting and emotional. Sharing other parents' personal stories from websites such as *All That Love Can Do* (www.allthatlovecando.blogspot.com), *Carrying to Term* (www.carryingtoterm.org), or *Sufficient Grace Ministries* (www.sufficientgraceministries.org), can be reaffirming and strength-building as she navigates the remainder of her time with her baby in her belly.

Emergency Scenarios: In some situations, when mom's life is compromised, parents do not have the luxury of time to make a decision. Parents who face this scenario feel additionally burdened. Amongst the chaos of an emergent situation, there is rarely time to consider creating memories when the only focus is saving mom's life. Depending on the gestation of baby, the sense of urgency for mom's safety and the type of procedure that will be performed, there are many variables to consider on a case-by-case basis.

- Offer information clearly
- Identify the procedure that she will be having
- Explain what to expect before, during, and after
- Request chaplain or clergy, if desired
- Be sensitive to the enormity of this decision and loss
- Make a recording of baby's heartbeat
- If possible, allow mom to hold baby
- If appropriate, capture baby's photo
- If given permission, create keepsakes for parents (see page 127, *Memory Making Options*)
- Schedule follow-up appointment before mom is discharged
- Send home with local and online resources
- Call to check on mom's physical and emotional healing

HELP NAVIGATE MEDICAL PROCESSES. ADVOCATE FOR FAMILIES NO MATTER THEIR DECISION.

Parents make the best decision with the information presented to them at the time. Many times, parents are surprised at the conclusion of their choice. Some parents who self-identify as pro-choice may decide to carry to term, while others who self-identify as pro-life may choose to end a much loved and wanted pregnancy. These decisions are well-thought, discussed, wrestled with, and agonized over. Both outcomes are devastating and heartbreaking to parents because neither outcome is one where their baby survives. No parent ever wants to make these horrific decisions. Every parent only wants to bring home a healthy, living baby.

As a health professional, your job is to educate, inform, and support your patients. There are times when the choice a patient makes will differ from your personal opinion or beliefs. Your patient cannot know this. When all information is relayed and a family has made the decision on how to proceed, they need your unconditional support. They will repeatedly need to hear that they are good parents and that their choice was made with love and is supported.

Even though parents have ultimately decided how to proceed, it does not mean that a family will feel relief about the outcome. The decision made merely means that out of two awful situations, they choose the lesser of the two for their family and their child. Many times, this decision haunts them, as one is never quite certain that the "right" choice was made. It is important that parents are given resources to support them. It is also helpful to refer parents to local or online support groups. Connecting with others who have had to make similar choices will ease their isolation.

EDUCATE THE FAMILY. PREPARE THEM FOR ALL OUTCOMES.

It is important to prepare families for all outcomes, including the possibility that baby may not survive. This conversation must be gentle, respectful, and direct, with the intention of support for healing. No family will ever be mentally or emotionally prepared for the death of their child, but knowing in advance that a child will not survive, families can be prepared to create memories and to know what to expect. When they learn that time is limited, preparations can be made.

Perinatal Hospice and Palliative Care: Perinatal hospice and palliative care is a model of compassionate care created for mom, baby, and the entire family. A tremendous amount of materials are available to ensure that families are offered tangible support while waiting to welcome and say goodbye to their baby. Although not a curative approach, the intention of perinatal hospice is to focus on comfort care and the quality of baby's life. Regardless of the length of time baby is alive, she is still entitled to a life of love, dignity, respect, and grace.

With your guidance, a care plan will be co-created specific to each individual family's needs. This practical guidance, as well as emotional/educational support, must begin at the time of discovery in pregnancy. It must also continue through labor and delivery, including life and the time after, when baby is no longer living. The plan that is created alongside the family will ensure they experience the least amount of regrets in such a devastating time. By having these difficult conversations before the actual moment, families are able to:

- Personalize a birth plan regardless of trimester
- Find a birth and bereavement doula
- Locate a remembrance family photographer
- Gather supplies for memory making
- Invite clergy for spiritual rites
- Ask about cultural practices or preferences
- Extend the invitation for family and/or friends to meet baby
- Include parents' other children in meeting baby, if desired
- Be informed of the physical appearance of baby upon delivery
- Prepare for the silence of stillbirth
- Decide to pursue life support or allow natural death
- Be educated on what to expect during the dying process
- Be offered options for neonatal organ donation
- Make mortuary arrangements

There are a tremendous number of hospitals adopting this protocol and many of them can be found at the *Perinatal Hospice & Palliative Care* website (www.perinatalhospice.org). If your hospital does not yet have a perinatal hospice and pediatric palliative care program, please utilize the the resource section (page 143), to guide the creation of your services. Utilizing this model of care can truly change the trajectory of a bereaved family's healing by reducing the amount of regret they experience.

The Labor & Delivery Process

**SLOW DOWN. BREATHE. ALLOW THE FAMILY TIME TO PROCESS
THE MAGNITUDE OF THEIR LOSS. THERE IS NO RUSH.**

If a baby will be born still, many moms will need the additional time to process what is about to happen. They may feel hesitant, terrified and ask for a caesarian. Explain to her that most often a vaginal delivery is the safest option with fewer risks and a more straightforward physical recovery. Also, it is important to share with her that many moms will feel an unexpected emotional release and sense of pride with the physical act of birthing their baby.

Unless medically necessary, do not rush mom to induce labor, do not rush her to deliver and do not rush her final moments of pregnancy. This news will take a lifetime to comprehend; allow her the grace to handle her labor and delivery as she wishes. She may want to go home to gather special items for baby. She may need fresh air to catch her breath. She may need to take a long bath and have her last precious moments with baby in her belly. Unless there is a need or mom's health is in danger, please allow her time.

When it is time for mom to labor, whether naturally or by induction, encourage her to express her wishes. Some birthing mothers want to numb the physical pain and will ask for an epidural. Other moms want to feel the physical pain as part of the grieving process to match their emotions. Do not assume to know what she wants. Do not insist that she do something other than her decision, unless it is against her best interests. You are the professional, help guide her.

These are the final moments that she has with baby in her belly, allow her to take time necessary to breathe. She has a huge task ahead to deliver, to meet and say goodbye to baby. Give her the space to mentally prepare as much as one possibly can in this situation.

ACKNOWLEDGE A BIRTHING MOTHER. CREATE A SAFE SPACE FOR HER TO DELIVER HER BABY.

Expecting mom to assimilate to the news that her baby has died and then expecting her to focus on delivering the baby she is carrying, is a tremendous amount of pressure. Our bodies carry stress in many different ways and it will take time for a mom to gather herself enough to do this impossible task. Even though her baby has died or will die, she is still baby's mother. She is still a mother in labor. Now, she is not only in physical pain, she is emotionally devastated.

It is important to create a space that will allow her to be as peaceful as can be. Offer chaplaincy services, while clearly explaining their non-denominational supportive role. If she has a trusted counselor or clergy member, invite them to speak or pray with her. If mom had a birth plan, remind her of it. If she planned on using a doula, encourage her to contact them. If she planned a photographer, ask a family member to call them. Allow her time to prepare for the event that lies ahead.

If mom requires medication to ease the anxiety of delivery, administer a dosage that allows her to be present and remember this brief time. She may not understand that she will want these memories in the future. Explain to her that while this time is utterly devastating, she will need to recount these moments later in life to process her grief, to remember and know her baby. This time, while excruciating, is part of her child's story. She will replay these moments over and over in her mind and you are facilitating healing for her future. Help her to remain calm so she can relax enough to deliver her baby.

BE PRESENT. TAKE TIME TO EXPLAIN AND PREPARE FAMILY FOR WHAT TO EXPECT. RESPECT THIS SACRED TIME.

Not knowing what to expect can be terrifying. It is not often that you will encounter a family that knows the intricacies of losing a baby, whether ending a wanted pregnancy, experiencing a stillbirth, carrying to term, or having a medically fragile, terminal baby. Each instance is scary and overwhelming to families.

Please share with families what to expect and do so slowly, kindly, calmly, and patiently. Be explicit but respectful when addressing what they will experience and see, remembering that this is their baby. While the medical term "fetal demise" is medically accurate, to mom and dad, this is their child.

- Speak slowly, clearly
- Be explicit in description
- Be sensitive in your words
- Take them through, step-by-step
- Allow parents' emotional response
- Ask for clarifying questions
- Answer all questions to the best of your ability, or find someone who can
- Repeat yourself as much as needed
- Continue to check in with parents
- Be available for questions later

SAY BABY'S NAME. WRITE BABY'S NAME. REFER TO MOM AND DAD AS BABY'S PARENTS.

Loving thought went into the naming of baby. Say baby's name. Every chance, say her name. The more you say baby's name, the more it will encourage family members to do the same. It will normalize speaking about baby. It will demonstrate how loved baby is. A baby's name, whether living or deceased, is the most beautiful word to parents.

- Learn how baby's name was chosen
- Write baby's name on the board in the room
- Write her name on the crib card
- Introduce parents as baby's (name) parents
- When referring to baby, always use her name

The Health Professional: Role & Impact

HAVING AN EMOTIONAL RESPONSE IS HUMAN.
IT'S OKAY TO SHOW YOUR EMOTIONS.

Showing emotions to a family allows them to see that they are not only a patient, but that their experience matters. Patients want to know that those tending to them truly care and that their personal loss is monumental.

In the short time a family has with their baby, typically only nurses, doctors, and social workers are amongst family to witness such a brief existence. It is a sacred time to be in the presence of a family's baby. These moments become life-long memories, so it's important to recognize it as such. If you are called to tears or any emotional response, allow that to be seen. The visual display of emotion validates the tremendous loss that the family is experiencing and anything other than expressing true human emotion feels cold. Show the family that their baby is real and important. Express to them your sadness for their loss.

CELEBRATE EVERY MILESTONE WITH PARENTS.
HELP CREATE HEALING EXPERIENCES.

If mom is on bed rest, chances are, you will come to know her pretty well. When a baby does not survive, memories of her hospital stay become baby's entire life. Although fast and fleeting, there are many milestones to be celebrated during the time when mom is waiting for the arrival of her baby. Celebrate the moments with her. She may not know to acknowledge these moments; do them for her, with her.

- Offer to take her weekly belly photo
- Learn how she chose baby's name
- Ask to hold her hand during procedures

And, when the moment comes that it is discovered that her baby has died or will not survive, reassure her that she will survive this loss in the most sensitive manner possible. Give her resources: a book, a pamphlet, a news article, a website — anything that gives her hope through the knowledge that others have survived this unimaginable loss. She trusts you as her caregiver, you are the professional. Be there for her in her sadness, too. When she delivers baby, be present. Don't stray or shy away from her. She shared her hope for baby, and now her most painful experience, with you. Share the loss with her. Be present and unafraid to talk to her.

ACKNOWLEDGE AND APPRECIATE ALL MOMENTS THE FAMILY HAS WITH BABY. YOU ARE THE MEMORY MAKERS.

For babies born with a life-limiting diagnosis and in the neonatal intensive care unit, there are, unfortunately, many reasons a parent may not be able to sit bedside. Although most parents do not ever want to leave their baby, at times, mom's medical needs, other children, or jobs may not allow parents to be in the NICU all hours of the day. This is a tremendously stressful time for families as they balance obligations that they cannot delegate.

In the times that parents are away, you are the memory makers. They may seem small and insignificant to you, but families will treasure any item that you create or gather for them in their absence. With permission:

- Take baby's photo
- Create a scrapbook page for parents
- Decorate isolette with baby's name
- Write messages in a children's book for baby
- Accept any donated items on behalf of parents (blanket, knit hat, etc.)

SHOW COMPASSION IN YOUR WORDS AND ACTIONS.
REMEMBER THAT THIS IS A LOVED AND WANTED CHILD.

This baby is the entire world to her parents. With the death of their child, their world has been destroyed. Every moment that a family has with their baby, whether in utero or after delivery, is the only time that they get in their entire life. Each interaction becomes an ingrained memory. Be aware of the impact every comment and action will have. Be compassionate. Be human. Be loving. Be kind. You have many opportunities to show compassion to families:

- Hold baby gently, affectionately, as you would a living child
- Ask baby's name. Use baby's name
- Upon birth or meeting baby, comment on baby's beauty and perfection
- Express sorrow for their tremendous loss
- Show emotion
- Ask for the honor to hold baby when it is time to say goodbye

CREATE MEMORABLE EXPERIENCES FOR THE FAMILY.
MAKE THE IMPOSSIBLE, POSSIBLE.

When encountering a family whose baby is on hospice, you have the unique opportunity to make the impossible a reality for them. Ask parents what wishes they have for their child and what they dreamt of experiencing with their baby. Obviously, their truest wish would be for their child to survive and be healthy, but since you cannot do that, be open to what wishes you can grant them. You will be surprised at the simplicity.

For some, being able to experience fresh air with their baby, take baby outside, feel the sun on her face, or watch the sunset together is a dream come true. For others, it may be to meet long distance family, to sit in the pool with their child, to play her the guitar. Be creative with how you can create these situations. Technology is so helpful — use it to your advantage.

These dreams, when they become reality, allow a small glimpse of normalcy and one less regret that a family will experience. As long as baby is safe and monitored, you can be a hero to a family by making the impossible possible and granting a simple wish.

TEND TO PARENTS, AS WELL AS BABY.
SUPPORT THE FAMILY FROM START TO FINISH.

It takes an incredible amount of energy and strength to endure the time leading up to and after experiencing the loss of a baby. The amount of emotional stress takes a toll on every part of the body. Sleep, appetite, and thirst are all affected.

Be sure to check in with the family and encourage them to take care of their physical needs. Chances are, they will put their needs last. Remind parents that in order to stay healthy and remain present, it is important to eat nourishing foods, remain hydrated, and try their best to rest during the day and sleep each night. This experience is a marathon, not a sprint, and they will need endurance to survive the emotional effects that last much longer than they expect.

- Remind parents to eat
- Make sure their water cup is always filled
- Encourage them to nap/sleep at night
- Inform them of patient support sites such as *CaringBridge* (www.caringbridge.org) and *Give InKind* (www.giveinkind.com)
- Create space in the hospital room for both mom and partner to rest comfortably

This support is needed throughout the time that their baby is living, but is also necessary to remember after their child has died. If parents are choosing to spend additional time with baby, it is still important for them to respond to their needs. Mom is recovering from delivery and needs to stay nourished and hydrated and her partner needs to keep his/her energy sustained to help tend to mom's physical needs.

CREATE A SACRED SPACE FOR THE FAMILY. YOU BECOME PART OF THEIR STORY, PART OF THEIR CHILD'S FAMILY.

The confines of the hospital can be stifling. The sounds, the smell, the other families in such close proximity can feel so overwhelming and distracting to families who want 100% of their focus on their child in this present moment.

Whether a family has experienced a stillbirth or is discontinuing life support, creating a sacred space for the family offers them respect and dignity for the enormity of this experience. If your hospital has the funding, creating a separate sacred space for grieving families is the most ideal scenario.

Be sure to include:

- Soft painted walls
- Natural lighting for remembrance photography
- Cuddle Cot™
- Crib
- Comfortable seating
  ◦ Large bed
  ◦ Sofa
  ◦ Oversized chair
  ◦ Rocking chair
- Soft blankets and pillows
- Reading materials (see page 136, *Resources*)
  ◦ *Navigating the Unknown: An Immediate Guide When Experiencing the Loss of Your Baby*, Amie Lands
  ◦ Stories of hope
  ◦ Books about grief

- ◦ Local resources
- Music Options
  - ◦ iPod dock & speaker
  - ◦ Stereo with CD's
- Memory boxes
  - ◦ Hand/foot imprints
  - ◦ Digital camera and memory card
- Play space for parents' living children
  - ◦ Crayons and coloring space
  - ◦ Rug to play on
  - ◦ Children's books
  - ◦ Toys
- Food/beverages
  - ◦ Fresh water
  - ◦ Snacks
  - ◦ Keurig with coffee and tea
- Essential Oils
  - ◦ Lavender, vetiver, rose, bergamot, ylang ylang, chamomile
  - ◦ Diffuser, roller ball, spritzer

You may not have the option for a complete bereavement room. Be creative. If possible, transfer the family to a separate room far from mothers with crying babies. If a private room is not possible, use the resources you have available. Make the family as comfortable as they can be given the constraints.

- Move the family to the farthest room/space in the department
- Play soft music or white noise
- Bring baby into bed with mom
- Offer extra pillows or a warm blanket
- Use a rocking chair to rock baby

- Put up extra privacy curtains
- Turn off the sound on baby's monitors
- Dim the lights
- Guide them through memory making with their baby (see page 127, *Memory Making Options*)
- Be the "keeper of the room"; block unwanted visitors and caution auxiliary staff before entering
- If possible, create a private space in the waiting room for the support group as well

BE FAMILIAR WITH NEONATAL ORGAN DONATION. HAVE RESOURCES AVAILABLE TO INFORM PARENTS OF THEIR OPTIONS.

Creating a legacy that extends beyond their baby's life can feel very comforting to a family. Many families are interested in infant organ donations but do not have the time or wherewithal to do research during their own personal tragedy. It is of great use for health professionals to be well-versed in organ donation so that they can respond to families when faced with their inquiries.

There are multiple types of donation for transplant, as well as for research, and each holds their own unique requirements. It is important to differentiate the types of donation, as well as the requirements that will need to be met so families can make an informed decision. They will need to understand timelines that must be followed for each type donation. They must also make choices, such as having their child returned to them after a recovery surgery, or if handing them over for the surgery will become their final goodbye.

Some families will want to proceed with organ donation despite the timelines mandated, but others may find those requirements dissuade them. It's important for families to be made aware of all details that this decision entails. Whatever choice a family makes is the right decision for them. It is important parents feel supported, regardless the outcome.

The Purposeful Gift (www.purposefulgift.com) was created as a result of one family's quest for organ donation for their infant son. This website shares user-friendly, organized information about organ, eye, tissue and whole body donation.

After Death

REDUCE FUTURE REGRETS. GUIDE FAMILIES TO SPEND QUALITY TIME WITH THEIR BABIES.

Your hospital may not have a space dedicated entirely to families experiencing loss, but that doesn't mean that you can't create a sacred space within their hospital room. It is important to note on the door that a grieving family resides inside, so that everyone who enters is aware.

While there are rituals and crafts that can be done to memorialize this time, it is so important to first give families the time and space to hold baby. They may be fearful to do so; they may decline seeing baby. Explain to them that many families have expressed the importance of meeting their child, to see, hold, and parent baby in the only time that they will have with her. It is your job to gently encourage them to eliminate what will be a possible regret in the future.

When parents are ready, handle baby as you would a living child. Help guide the family through this time. Teach parents how to swaddle her and be respectful as you hand her over to parents. Have parents note the weight of baby in their arms and against their chest. Encourage them to unravel the hospital blanket and adore the beautiful child that they created, that grew in mom's body. Show them baby's fingers, toes, the folds of her ear. Find any birthmarks or "angel" kisses, and any similarities between baby and mom or dad.

The act of parenting baby is so empowering. Parents have no way of knowing how impactful these moments will become in the future.

STRATEGIES FOR HEALTH PROFESSIONALS

Encourage each partner to hold baby for as long as they are comfortable. For some parents, that will be minutes, for others, it could be hours. There is no rushing this time that they cannot get back.

- Model how to bathe baby
- Offer parents the chance to diaper baby
- Support the desire to dress baby in a planned outfit or in one that the hospital is able to supply
- Teach how to swaddle baby

PHOTOGRAPHS ARE IRREPLACEABLE.
THEY ARE TREASURED BEYOND MEASURE.

A bereaved parent gets a finite amount of time with their baby; these moments cannot be revisited and they cannot be replaced. Parents may think that they will remember every last detail about their baby, but that just isn't so. Grief, exhaustion and time wears on the memory and these photographs become prized possessions. These photographs can provide tremendous comfort in the future. Whether families choose to use a professional service or take photographs with their own cameras or cell phones, these photographs validate the existence and presence of these precious moments.

Families may deny the opportunity to have photographs taken because it feels unnatural. They may fear what others think or assume they won't want to remember baby in this state. In most cases, those concerns are unfounded.

If the parents seem hesitant, take the time to explain that other families have found photos to bring significant comfort in the days to come. As hard as it is to see the result of their child not living, a parent's love for their child is stronger than anything the eyes may see. Having a photograph to share with siblings and other family members will be meaningful to those that were not able to be there. One of the largest regrets for many families is their wish to have had taken photos of and with their child. Gently insist that parents take photos or invite a photographer, even if they think they will never look at them. It's better to have the photos safely stored at home and never looked at, than have a parent regret their entire life the missed opportunity to have these pictures.

Now I Lay Me Down to Sleep (USA) and Heartfelt (AU) are two non-profit organizations that offer remembrance photography at no cost to families. They work with professional photographers worldwide and they believe that these images serve as an important step in the family's healing process through honoring the child's legacy. The photos are tastefully edited and lovingly prepared for families. Volunteer photographers are vetted and professionally trained to interact with families during this loss. They are kind, respectful, and serve as a valuable resource.

If for some reason a photographer is not available, with the family's permission, please take photos of baby yourself. There are so many fine details that parents will want to remember. Be sure to take all the photos as you would any newborn baby. Capture the sweetness of her body: fingers, toes, ears, chin, nose, eyelashes, and any hair on her head. Be sure to include both parents in the pictures with her: holding her, kissing her, each parent holding her alone and the family as a whole. If any other family members are there, include them, even the children. Leave no photo idea unsnapped. This is the one chance to capture every moment of their time with baby. Take advantage of the time available, for as long as you feel inclined.

Photo Checklist:
- clothed
- nude
- in diaper
- hands
- fingers

- feet
- toes
- chin
- nose
- lips
- ears
- eyelashes
- hair
- baby bottom
- being held
- in bassinet
- on scale, showing weight
- with special items
- with entire family
- with mom: holding, faces close, kissing, adoring baby
- with dad: holding, faces close, kissing, adoring baby
- with siblings: parent holding baby, siblings adoring baby, individual siblings holding baby
- with grandparents or guests: holding, kissing

All moments are perfect opportunities for a photographer to capture. Whether families have a professional photographer, a non-profit volunteer, a digital camera, or smartphone, be sure to take the photos. The pictures need not be posed. Lifestyle moments will capture true emotions and will be treasured later when memories fail them.

CREATE MEMORIAL ITEMS WITH THE FAMILY.

There are many memories that a family can make with their child, whether baby was born living or born still. Some families are uncomfortable with this thought, or think that they do not want to interrupt this valuable time by doing "arts and crafts". But this is the only time that they will have with their baby. The time that they get to hold their child is far less than it was ever supposed to be. Once they hand their baby over for the last time, that is it. They don't get that time back, but they can hold those keepsakes for the rest of their lives.

It is important to initiate a dialogue about memory making. In doing so, you are helping to reduce regrets that the family could potentially experience in the future. An open and continued conversation with parents will help to understand their position, cultural preferences, and spiritual beliefs, while possibly dispelling any fears and concerns they may have. When a family is in the midst of such devastation and trauma, they may be unable to see the value in these items and fear may hold them back. Families may be unaware of the options available and when they do realize them, it is often too late. By discussing together and supporting their decision, you are softening the blunt force that this grief will bestow upon them.[1]

Memory making can help facilitate healthy grieving. These keepsakes provide a tangible gift and precious memories of parenting their baby. Regardless if parents think they will or will not want these items in the future, it is better to have them and never use them than not have them at all. Research has shown that families who have met, bathed, dressed and spent time with their baby are better able to cope in the healing process; it helps the brain comprehend what has happened and the activities allow the parent to create memories they otherwise wouldn't have.[2]

This is a sacred time, holding one's child in the space between this life and next — treat it as such. It can be terrifying for parents, not

1 Adzich, K., Davis, D., Hochberg, T., Kavanaugh, K., Kobler, K., Lammert, C. A., . . . Press, J. N. (2016). Pregnancy Loss and Infant Death Alliance (PLIDA) position statement on offering the baby to bereaved parents with relationship-base care (Rev. ed.). Retrieved from the PLIDA website: http://www.plida.org/position-statements/
2 Institute of Medicine (US) Committee on Palliative and End-of-Life Care for Children and Their Families; Field, M.J., Behrman, R.E., editors. When Children Die: Improving Palliative and End-of-Life Care for Children and Their Families. Washington (DC): National Academies Press (US); 2003. APPENDIX E, BEREAVEMENT EXPERIENCES AFTER THE DEATH OF A CHILD

knowing what to expect. They may have never seen a person after death and the unknown can be overwhelming. Remind them that this is their baby. They created this perfect being and she will always be perfect to them. Each moment they choose to spend with baby will be treasured for the rest of their lives, even if it is the most painful of times. Show them their baby was more than a patient, show them their baby was loved, valued and will always be important.

Memory Making Options:
- Take photos
- Bathe baby
- Change diaper
- Dress baby
- Swaddle baby
- Stamps, imprints, 3-D molds
- Cut a lock of hair
- Keepsakes; hospital bracelet, card with weight, etc.

Depending on indiviual circumstances, some families will not have the opportunity to create memorial items with their baby. If after discussing with parents, the family has expressed interest and granted permission for keepsakes but does not want (or is unable) to be present for their creation, please create these items for them. Things such as hand/footprints, imprints and molds can be of such comfort when the family has returned home.

Stamps: In addition to the footprints traditionally taken by hospital staff upon a live birth, please take handprints as well. Ask the family if they want more than one stamp, or if they want to include siblings with baby's prints side-by-side. Some parents later use these stamps as the foundation of art projects in their home with pre-existing or future children, and some even use them as tattoos. Upon returning home, it is extremely important that they are instructed to make a copy of these prints to avoid losing them to fading in future years.

Imprints: Hand and foot imprints are the next step up from a stamped print. Imprints are made from a clay-like substance that will harden over time, giving a realistic imprint of baby's hands and fingers, their tiny feet and their sweet little toes. This is moderately gentle for baby's skin and can later be painted or sealed with spray paint to help it last over time.

Molds: 3-D molds are actual 3-D replicas that are created by sticking baby's hand and/or foot into a mold kit purchased from a craft store. The 3-D mold is amazing in its authenticity to the child's actual hand and foot. You can see every nook, cranny, fingerprint and hand-line. A family can hold a replica of their child's actual foot in the palm of their hand when baby is no longer with them.

This process is less delicate and will not do well if the infant died before birth. You, the professional, will have to be the judge to know if using a 3-D mold is appropriate for baby's skin. Also, 3-D molds are a bit temperamental to create. Be sure to have practice with this craft and ask for assistance when performing this task, either by another staff member or a family member, if they are comfortable.

When the family returns home, similar to the imprints, they will need to be sure to seal or paint the molds so that they survive the elements that could erode or fade them over time. A sealing spray paint will be sufficient to seal the porous material of the mold.

Keepsakes: Many families want to gather keepsakes from their child to put in a baby book, or a special box. Among these items, families have chosen to include the crib card, photos, hospital bracelets, locks of hair and other memorabilia. For some, collecting and creating these items may be against their beliefs or wishes, so you must have a conversation before doing so. Be certain to only gather items for which you have been granted permission.

While in the hospital, be sure families take great care to store these items safely in a special place until they can find a permanent spot in their home. They won't regret making these mementos and, someday, may find themselves longing for them if they choose not to create them.

PARENTING CONTINUES BEYOND LIFE. ENCOURAGE TIME TO SAY GOODBYE. THESE MOMENTS CANNOT BE RETURNED.

When baby has died, there are moments after death that a parent would never know to consider. In the movies, we see family members leave the room as soon as a death occurs, but in real life, there are tremendous opportunities for healing rituals to take place. Although they may initially feel apprehensive, families may be open to having you guide them through various acts as they prepare for their final good-bye. Most importantly, remind parents to breathe, stay present, trust their instincts, and follow their heart. Suggest that families:

- Light a candle
- Talk to baby
- Sing to baby
- Read baby a children's book
- Pray or give blessings over baby's body
- Play music
- Bathe baby
- Memorize baby's body before dressing her
- Dress baby in her finest outfit and/or swaddle baby
- Take lots of photos (refer to page 124, *Photo Checklist*)
- Hold baby as long as they want
- Invite friends and family to meet baby
- Take baby home before cremation or burial, where legal

Give the family as much time as they want and need with their baby. They are fitting an entire lifetime into these moments. For some families, the time they spend with baby after death may be minutes.

For others, it might be hours or even days — when possible, with the use of a Cuddle Cot™ or a cooling system. Encourage the family to take their time and insist that there is no pressure to rush these moments.

When it is time, and the family is ready to hand baby over for the last time, that moment is so important. Do not take it lightly. The words you say and the actions you take will forever be the final memory that a family has with their baby.

- It is **your honor** to hold their baby
- Assure them you will take good care of their baby
- Hold baby as if she were a living child
- Be respectful as you leave the room
- If possible, hold baby as you leave
- If not possible, use a bassinet adorned with a blanket

Your gentle presence will be a lifelong treasured memory. You will have met, cared for, and known their baby. Not many in the world will have had that privilege.

Re-entering the World Without Baby

GIVE PARENTS IMPORTANT INFORMATION IN EVERY WAY POSSIBLE. BE PREPARED WITH REFERRALS AND RESOURCES FOR WHEN THE FAMILY RETURNS HOME.

It is important to give families support as they enter the grief experience by offering resources that foster healing. Have materials prepared for families so that all the information they need is in one location for later reference. Include reading material, counseling services, support groups (online and in person), and educational information about pursuing a subsequent pregnancy, should they show interest. Share retreats to connect with other bereaved families, opportunities for remembrance events, and contacts to create memorial items.

For every situation that health professionals encounter, there are a multitude of resources that can help guide families, including educational materials, professional support, peer support, retreats, memorial items, and remembrance opportunities. Within your practice, have resources prepared for any and all situations so that when you are faced with a patient experiencing any type loss, you can easily locate and offer them correct information. Be certain to include with your bereavement materials, information regarding postpartum healing and options to donate breast milk or cease lactation when mom's milk comes in.

Grieving the death of one's child is isolating and family and friends often do not have the words or capacity to ease the pain of this loss. Having support from other bereaved parents who understand the depth of grief can be a true comfort. There are countless opportunities for parents to connect with others. Online sites such as *Still Standing* (www.stillstandingmag.com), *Still Mothers* (www.stillmothers.com), and *Glow in the Woods* (www.glowinthewoods.com) can offer support in the safety of one's home. Healing retreats such as the Return to Zero Center for Healing, Faith's Lodge, and Selah: MISS Foundation Retreat provide irreplaceable bonding experiences for families to connect with one another while receiving professional support for healing.

Give parents more information than you think they may need — more information is better than not enough. They will likely have many questions, but some thoughts may come later after they have settled in at home. Be sure to include contact information for someone parents can call when they have the strength and clarity to talk after processing this loss. Do not send families home empty handed. Know your local resources. Direct them to in-person support, as well as online services for the times that they do not feel capable of leaving home. Support is necessary to healing and peer support is invaluable.

OFFER A WEIGHTED ITEM. GIVE EMPTY ARMS
SOMETHING TANGIBLE TO HOLD.

The devastation as a family leaves the hospital without their baby is traumatizing. Parents will tell you that their arms physically ache to hold their baby. This phenomena is so widespread, it is being preliminarily researched by the Institute for Palliative Medicine at the San Diego Hospice in California, USA. When offered the use of a weighted teddy bear called The Comfort Cub® bereaved mothers found that "being able to embrace this infant-sized object in her arms led to profound relief".[3]

The idea of filling empty arms is so important. There are many organizations to choose from. Some weighted items are created with a generic weight, while others will customize the weight to exactly that of baby at birth. There are do-it-yourself directions to create these at home, as well. And while it is most ideal to receive this during the hospital stay, having the resources available for families to independently pursue a weighted item of their choice can also be of assistance. Many families have more than one in their home. Some have one for each parent. Others even include having a weighted item for siblings. The positive impact that these can have in healing is significant.

HELP FAMILIES REMEMBER THEIR BABIES. CREATE, PARTICIPATE,
OR REFER FAMILIES TO LOCAL REMEMBRANCE EVENTS.

Remembrance events offer incredible opportunities for professional and peer support. These events allow parents to reconnect with the professionals who cared for their baby and also connect (often for the first time) with other bereaved parents. Not only does it provide space for their baby to be honored, it reduces isolation for the parents so they

3 Institute for Palliative Medicine at the San Diego Hospice. CA. (US); Johnson, M. Bruckner, T., Moore, S., M.D., M.P.H., Ferris, F.D., M.D., FAAHPM; The Therapeutic Use and Impact of The Comfort Cub® Program In Perinatal Bereavement

can see they are not alone in their grief. At a remembrance event, there are many simple ways to honor a baby who has died:

- Light candles
- Release butterflies
- Play music
- Offer a craft activity
- Say each baby's name aloud during the service
- Have baby's name printed in the written program

Pregnancy and Infant Loss Remembrance Day on October 15, and the Annual Worldwide Candle Lighting each second Sunday of December, provide the perfect opportunity to create organized events in which to invite, gather, and support bereaved families. These internationally recognized dates encourage others to support bereaved families by acknowledging them, their child, and their loss.

HONOR EACH BABY, THEIR LIFE AND THEIR MEMORY.
BE COMPASSIONATE, KIND, CARING, AND HONEST.

As time moves on, many families' largest worry after their baby has died is that their child will be forgotten. There are many gestures to demonstrate that their baby is remembered. These offerings create a lasting impression and are truly appreciated:

- Send a condolence card shortly after returning home
- Send an annual card for baby's birthday or anniversary
- Donate to an organization in memory of baby on behalf of the staff

By creating opportunities in which to acknowledge a family's baby, you are saying without words, "Your baby is important, is valued, and will always be remembered." Because these babies are important, valued, and will always be remembered — let it be known to her parents.

Take Care of Your Heart

Your job is tremendous. The weight that you carry and the human condition that you bear witness to is a huge burden to shoulder. Take gentle care of your heart, too.

While this is a day at work for you, it is life-altering for your patient. The way in which you interact with them and care for their baby will forever be the greatest gift. Before entering the room of a patient experiencing loss, take a few minutes to get centered. For their entire life, they will appreciate the emotional presence you offer.

When your shift is over, do something kind for yourself. Release the heavy emotions that you have carried your entire day and know that you did your very best for your patient, her baby, and her family. Breathe, cry, take a shower, hydrate, eat nourishing food, and be in the presence of whatever fuels your soul. Your job is greater than "going to work". Your job is the first step in a very long journey of grief. But, with your loving kindness, your care can offer the first steps toward healing.

Resources

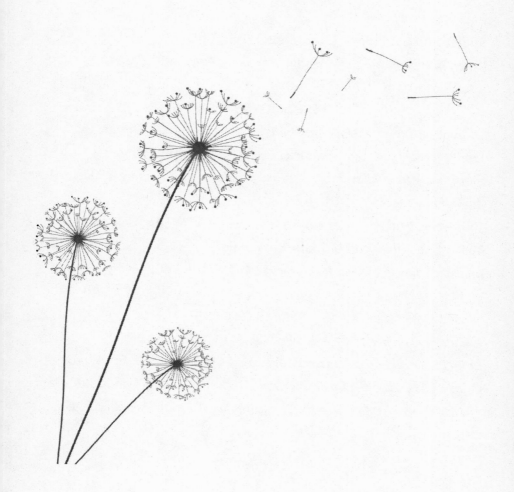

Support Books

IMMEDIATE SUPPORT

Navigating the Unknown: An Immediate Guide When Experiencing the Loss of Your Baby, Amie Lands

A Gift of Time, Amy Kuebelbeck and Deborah L. Davis, PhD

Empty Cradle, Broken Heart: Surviving the Death of Your Baby, Deborah L. Davis, PhD

Loving and Letting Go: For Parents Who Decided to Turn Away from Aggressive Medical Intervention for Their Critically Ill Newborns, Deborah L. Davis, PhD

Stillbirth, Yet Still Born, Deborah L. Davis, PhD

Unexpected Goodbye: When Your Baby Dies, Angela Rodman

SPECIFIC TO MOMS

Dear Cheyenne: A Journey Into Grief, Joanne Cacciatore, PhD

From Mother to Mother: On the Loss of a Child, Emily Long

Sunshine After the Storm: A Survival Guide for the Grieving Mother, Alexa Bigwarfe

You Are Not Alone: Love Letters From Loss Mom to Loss Mom, Emily Long

You Are the Mother of All Mothers, Angela Miller

Invisible Mothers: When Love Doesn't Die, Emily Long

SPECIFIC TO DADS

A Guide for Fathers: When a Baby Dies, Tim Nelson

From Father to Father: Letters From Loss Dad to Loss Dad, Emily Long

Grieving Dads: To the Brink and Back, Kelly Farley and David DiCola

The Griefcase: A Man's Guide To Healing and Moving Forward In Grief, R. Glenn Kelly

HEALTH PROFESSIONALS

Companioning at a Time of Perinatal Loss: A Guide for Nurses, Physicians, Social Workers, Chaplains and Other Bedside Caregivers, Jane Huestis, RN and Marcia Jenkins, RN

Grieving Beyond Gender: Understanding the Ways Men and Women Mourn, Kenneth J. Doka and Terry L. Martin

Time to Care: How to Love Your Patients and Your Job, Robin Youngson

Relationship-Based Care: A Model for Transforming Practice, Mary Koloroutis

Perinatal and Pediatric Bereavement in Nursing and Other Health Professions, Beth Perry Black, Patricia Moyle Wright, and Rana Limbo

MEMOIRS

A Piece of My Heart, Molly Fumia

An Exact Replica of a Figment of My Imagination, Elizabeth McCracken

Brona: A Memoir, Mara Hill

Expecting Adam, Martha Beck

Ghostbelly, Elizabeth Heineman

Holding Silvan, Monica Wesolowska

I Will Carry You, Angie Smith

Silvie's Life, Dr. Marianne Rogoff

The Lessons of Love, Melody Beattie

Waiting With Gabriel, Amy Kuebelbeck

What I Gave to the Fire, Kim Flowers Evans

PREGNANCY AFTER LOSS

Celebrating Pregnancy Again, Franchesca Cox

Expecting Sunshine, Alexis Marie Chute

Joy at the End of the Rainbow: A Guide to Pregnancy After a Loss, Amanda Ross-White

Pregnancy After a Loss, Carol Cirulli Lanham

GRIEF

A Broken Heart Still Beats: After Your Child Dies, Anne McCracken

Bearing the Unbearable: Love, Loss, and the Heartbreaking Path of Grief, Joanne Cacciatore, PhD

Dear Parents: Letters to Bereaved Parents, Centering Corporation

For Bereaved Grandparents, Margaret H. Gerner

Grief … Reminders for Healing, Gale Massey

Grieving Parents: Surviving Loss as a Couple, Nathalie Himmelrich

Permission to Mourn: A New Way to Do Grief, Tom Zuba

Surviving My First Year of Child Loss, Nathalie Himmelrich

The Grief Recovery Handbook, John W. James and Russell Friedman

Three Minus One: Stories of Parents' Love and Loss, Sean Hanish and Brooke Warner

Understanding Your Grief: Ten Essential Touchstones for Finding Hope and Healing Your Heart, Alan D. Wolfelt

When Children Grieve, John W. James and Russell Friedman with Dr. Leslie Landon Matthews

CHILDREN'S BOOKS

Healing Your Grieving Heart for Kids: 100 Practical Ideas, Alan D. Wolfelt

I Miss You: A First Look at Death, Pat Thomas

Lifetimes: The Beautiful Way to Explain Death to Children, Bryan Mellonie and Robert Ingpen

Someone Came Before You, Pat Schwiebert

Special Delivery, Melanie Tioleco-Cheng

Tear Soup: A Recipe for Healing After Loss, Pat Schwiebert and Chuck DeKlyen

The Invisible String, Patrice Karst and Geoff Stevenson

The Next Place, Warren Hanson

Turned Upside Down, Teana Tache

When Someone Dies: A Child-Caregiver Activity Book, National Alliance for Grieving Children

JOURNALS

Family Lasts Forever: A Very Special Baby Book, Noelle K. Andrew and Sheila B. Frascht

Life Without the Baby Journal: Redefining Life, Self, and Motherhood After Loss, Emily Long

Love Lasts Forever: A Journal of Memories, Noelle K. Andrew and Sheila B. Frascht

On Coming Alive: Journaling Through Grief, Lexi Behrndt

PHILOSOPHY, PSYCHOLOGY, SPIRITUAL, INSPIRATIONAL

A Deep Breath of Life: Daily Inspiration for Heart Centered Living, Alan Cohen

A Grief Observed, C.S. Lewis

Brave Enough, Cheryl Strayed

Broken Open: How Difficult Times Can Help Us Grow, Elizabeth Lesser

Healing After Loss: Daily Meditations for Working Through Grief, Martha Whitmore Hickman

Healing Through the Dark Emotions: The Wisdom of Grief, Fear and Despair, Miriam Greenspan

Heaven is for Real, Todd Burpo and Lynn Vincent

Life Prayers: From Around the World, Elizabeth Roberts and Elias Amidon

Option B: Facing Adversity, Building Resilience, and Finding Joy, Sheryl Sandberg and Adam Grant

Something Like Magic: On Remembering How to be Alive, Brian Andreas

The Power of a Broken-Open Heart: Life-Affirming Wisdom from the Dying, Julie Interrante, MA

The Untethered Soul: The Journey Beyond Yourself, Michael A. Singer

To Bless the Space Between Us, John O'Donohue

When Bad Things Happen to Good People, Harold S. Kushner

Who Dies? An Investigation of Conscious Living and Conscious Dying, Stephen and Ondrea Levine

Websites

AFTER DEATH ARRANGEMENTS

Association of Organ Procurement www.aopo.org

Cuddle Cot™ www.flexmort.com/cuddle-cots

Institute for the Advancement of Medicine Neonatal Donation Program www.iiam.org/

Purposeful Gift www.purposefulgift.com

AUTOPSY

Regional Pathology and Autopsy Services www.regional-pathology.com/faq

UF Health FAQs: Autopsy www.pathlabs.ufl.edu/services/autopsy/faq-autopsy

BURIAL GOWNS

Emma and Evan Foundation www.evefoundation.org

NICI Helping Hands www.nicuhelpinghands.org/programs/angel-gown-program

INFERTILITY

Still Mothers www.stillmothers.com/resources/infertility-resources

MEMORIAL ITEMS

Comfort Cub www.thecomfortcub.com

HEALing Embrace www.healingembrace.org

Illuminate Photography Course www.berylaynyoung.com/illuminate

Molly Bears www.mollybears.com

National Star Registry www.starregistry.com

Refuge in Grief Writing Course
www.refugeingrief.com/support/30-day
Seashore of Remembrance
www.theseashoreofremembrance.blogspot.com.au
The Story of...books www.thestoryof-books.com

MEMORY MAKING

Heartfelt www.heartfelt.org.au
Now I Lay Me Down to Sleep Posing Guide for Hospitals
www.nowilaymedowntosleep.org/medical/posing-guide-for-hospitals
Regali Silver Fingerprint Charms
www.regalijewelry.com/pages/hospitalshospices.php

MORTUARY/FUNERAL ARRANGEMENTS

Funeral Consumers Alliance www.funerals.org
Funerals vs. Celebration of Life
www.johnsonsfuneralhome.com/Funerals_vs._Celebrations_of_Life_1263241.html
Home Funerals Grow as American's Skip the Mortician for After Death Care
www.huffingtonpost.com/2013/01/25/home-funerals-death-mortician_n_2534934.html
Is there a difference between funeral home and a mortuary?
www.sciencecare.com/blog-is-there-a-difference-between-funeral-home-and-a-mortuary
National Home Funeral Alliance www.homefuneralalliance.org
Planning a Funeral or Memorial Service
www.sevenponds.com/after-death/planning-a-funeral-or-memorial-service

What is the Difference between a mortuary and a funeral home? www.imortuary.com/blog/what-is-the-difference-between-a-mortuary-and-a-funeral-home

ONLINE RESOURCES & EMOTIONAL SUPPORT

Compassionate Friends www.compassionatefriends.org

Facets of Grief www.facetsofgrief.com

Faces of Loss, Faces of Hope www.facesofloss.com

Glow in The Woods www.glowinthewoods.com

HAND, Helping After Neonatal Death www.handonline.org

National Alliance for Grieving Children www.childrengrieve.org

Pregnancy Loss and Infant Death Alliance www.PLIDA.org

Reconceiving Loss www.reconceivingloss.com

Share Pregnancy & Infant Loss Support www.nationalshare.org

Shared Grief Project www.sharedgrief.org

Star Legacy Foundation www.starlegacyfoundation.org

Still Mothers www.stillmothers.com

Still Standing Magazine www.stillstandingmag.com

The Grief Recovery Method www.griefrecoverymethod.com

The MISS Foundation www.missfoundation.org

The Ruthie Lou Foundation www.ruthieloufoundation.org

Unspoken Grief www.unspokengrief.com

PATIENT SUPPORT SITES

CarePages www.carepages.com

CaringBridge www.caringbridge.org

Give InKind www.giveinkind.com

Plumfund www.plumfund.com

YouCaring www.youcaring.com

PEDIATRIC PALLIATIVE CARE FACILITIES

George Mark Children's House www.georgemark.org

Ryan House www.ryanhouse.org

PERINATAL HOSPICE & PALLIATIVE CARE

Center to Advance Palliative Care
www.capc.org/topics/pediatric-palliative-care

End of Life Content in Treatment Guidelines for Life-Limiting Diseases
www.ncbi.nlm.nih.gov/pubmed/15684843

Focus on the Family
www.focusonthefamily.com/lifechallenges/relationship-challenges/when-your-baby-wont-survive/carrying-your-baby-to-term

Get Palliative Care www.getpalliativecare.org

Information About Serious Illness
www.baylorhealth.com/SiteCollectionDocuments/Documents_BHCS/BHCS_Patient%20Info_DocumentsForms/SeriousIllness_rev8.pdf

International Children's Palliative Care Network www.icpcn.org

National Hospice and Palliative Care Organization
www.nhpco.org/pediatric

Pediatric Palliative Care www.getpalliativecare.org/whatis/pediatric

Perinatal Hospice & Palliative Care List of Programs
www.perinatalhospice.org/list-of-programs

Perinatal Hospice & Palliative Care Resources for Caregivers
www.perinatalhospice.org/resources-for-caregivers

PREGNANCY OPTIONS

A Heartbreaking Choice www.aheartbreakingchoice.com

All That Love Can Do www.allthatlovecando.blogspot.com

Carrying to Term www.carryingtoterm.org

Ending a Wanted Pregnancy www.endingawantedpregnancy.com

8

Little Love Foundation www.littlelovefoundation.blogspot.com/p/fatal-diagnosis

Perinatal Hospice & Palliative Care www.perinatalhospice.org

Stillbirthday www.stillbirthday.com

Sufficient Grace Ministries www.sufficientgraceministries.org

RETREATS

Faith's Lodge www.faithslodge.org

Landon's Legacy Retreat www.landonslegacyretreat.com

Respite Retreat www.nancyguthrie.com/respite-retreat

Return to Zero Center for Healing
www.returntozerohealingcenter.com

Selah: MISS Foundation Retreat www.missfoundation.org

About the Contributors

ADRIEN MCGOON is a wife and the mother of five children: two angel boys, Henry and Emmett, a foster-adopt son, Owen, an adopted daughter, Hazel, and a bio son, Ronin. Adrien lives in northern California with her husband, Kevin, and has recently become a full-time momma.

ALEXA BIGWARFE is a wife, mother of three, dog owner, and advocate for those without a voice. She started blogging as an outlet for her grief after the loss of one of her twin daughters to Twin-to-Twin Transfusion Syndrome (TTTS) and now uses the blog to advocate for those without a voice (katbiggie.com). She has written/or edited and self-published numerous books of her own and for other authors through her hybrid publishing company, Kat Biggie Press. She uses that hard-earned publishing knowledge to support other writers and small businesses in completing, publishing, and marketing their books through her company Write.Publish.Sell (writepublishsell.co). She spends her free time writing about children's and maternal health topics and survival strategies for busy moms.

ANGELA OLSEN lives in Sonoma County, CA with her husband and daughter, and 3 angel babies watching over them. Angela works as a medical assistant, birth doula, lactation specialist, beauty consultant with Mary Kay Cosmetics and a childbirth educator. Affectionately known as the "Mary Kay doula", she enjoys working with women through education and empowerment. She enjoys spending time with her family, gardening, meditating, reading, teaching, and training. For more information please visit www.joyfuljourneybirthservices.com.

ANNE SHAMIYEH is a middle school teacher studying to become a nurse. She enjoys volunteering at UCSF Benioff Children's Hospital as a parent mentor in the intensive care nursery, helping to support other families through long NICU stays. It brings her joy to honor her son Kai, who spent his short six months of life at UCSF. She lives in San Francisco with her husband, Omar, and their daughters, Zara and Malia.

ANNELISE BOGE is a wife and mother of two babies in heaven, Annika and Andrew. She works as a pediatric occupational therapist in Reno, NV and enjoys gardening, reading, and spending time with her husband and their golden retriever, Dexter.

BETHANY CONKEL is the mommy to three amazing children, one who lives in heaven and two who live on earth. She is also an author, inspirational speaker, bereavement/comfort doula, bereavement photographer, and the founder of a non-profit organization called Purposeful Gift. Bethany's book, *A Momma's Heart: Comfort for Loss Moms*, was published in the fall of 2017, five years after the loss of her son. She has also written articles featured on *Yahoo!*, *The Mighty, and All That Love Can Do*. Bethany is passionate about neonatal donation, as her son was a research-exclusive organ and whole-body donor. She has used her experience to help other mothers and to inspire donation professionals. Bethany also serves with Sufficient Grace Ministries as a comfort doula and bereavement photographer. She resides in Ohio with her wonderful husband, Eric, and their daughters.

BLANDINE DE COINCY is a clinical psychologist who lives outside Paris, France. She is a wife and a mother of five beautiful children: two boys and two girls who can run, one daughter who can fly. After Sixtine's stillbirth, Blandine created and runs a retreat for bereaved parents all over France and Belgium (www.retraite-renaitre.com). She also participates in organizing an annual October 15th march in Paris to honor all the babies who departed earth too early.

BRILEY STIFFLER-WEIR is a registered nurse in the labor and delivery unit. While pursuing the dream of becoming a mom herself, Briley supported expecting moms before, during, and after the births of their babies. Previously a perinatal and infertility nurse coordinator, she has been witness to both the joy of welcoming new life and the sorrow of life not lived. Briley currently resides in Sonoma County, CA where she was raised and is now raising a family of her own.

DANIELLE SALINGER is finding herself, with humor and wit, through speaking her truths and facing her fears. She lives in northern California with her husband and daughter. She began writing about living with depression and anxiety, as well as adventures at home and other musings, and found that her honesty, sensitivity, and vulnerability struck a cord and inspired others. After the losses of her sons, Josiah in 2015 and Lincoln in 2017, she also began to write about pregnancy loss and grief, and started a blog for her thoughts at www. beingrealwithdanielle.com.

GAIL WHETSTINE lives in San Diego, CA with her husband, Alan. She is a mother of two angels, Heighley and Matthew. They have been blessed with two beautiful daughters, Lindsay and Chelsea. She is happiest when she is spending time with her two precious granddaughters, extending hospitality to family and friends, engaged in weekly Bible study and meditation groups, and taking long walks on the beach.

HEATHER BROWNE lives right outside Washington D.C. in northern Virginia. She is an educator, skincare consultant, advocate, wife, and mom to her three boys (two sunshine children and one angel baby).

She worked for over a decade as a high school English teacher and now coordinates an international program in a local high school. She also supports inner beauty through life-changing skincare, fiercely advocates for women's rights, and spends her free time with her friends and a household of active boys. Whatever she's doing, she does it with passion.

JACQUI MORTON lives in Massachusetts where she enjoys dance parties and pizza night with her husband and two favorite sons. She works as a writer, facilitator, and reproductive advocate. Jacqui is the author of a chapbook of poetry, *Turning Cozy Dark*, and has published work in places such as *Salon, the Guardian, MUTHA Magazine,* and *The Rumpus.* In 2015, she created Holding Our Space, a project that seeks to create spaces where folks can be open about their reproductive experiences, including abortion. She co-facilitates an annual retreat for women who have terminated a wanted pregnancy. Visit her at www.jacquimorton. com.

JESSICA McCOY is a mother of two children, one living boy and one stardust girl. She works at a domestic violence shelter and also as a doula. Her passion is supporting women and children, through all walks of life. She enjoys hiking, practicing yoga, writing, and spending time with her family and is located in Springfield, MO.

JESSICA MEYERS is a wife and mother of two wild boys, and a little girl who danced her way into eternity after spending 120 days earthside. She currently resides in the Pacific northwest with her husband and spends her days writing, creating memories with her sons, and finding moments full of her daughter.

JO-ANNE JOSEPH is a career woman, dreamer, artist, writer, and poet from South Africa. She is married to her best friend, Brian, and is, above all, a mother to two beautiful children: Braydon, with whom she gets to share her days and watch grow, and Zia, whom she holds in her heart. Love is what drives her to do more and do better for her family and for the loss community every day. She writes regularly for *Glow in the Woods* and *Still Standing Magazine* and is author of her debut book, *Infinity*, a contemporary romance novel. She is an avid reader and loves all things bookish, as well as time with her boys and expressing her heart in words.

KATIE WARD, mama to Liam, whose time on earth was far too brief, lives in northern California with her husband Brit and dog, Goose. She owns her own personal styling and mobile clothing business, which is run from her home. Katie enjoys reading, exercising, traveling and most of all, sharing the memory of Liam with others.

LAUREN LANE is a mom to three children, entering the world of loss after the stillbirth of her first daughter Rhiannon at 39 weeks from a cord accident/cord compression in March of 2013, following years of infertility. She is also mom to two living children and is a trauma therapist. She focuses her professional work on families and parents who have experienced infertility and the loss of a child, and writes for *Still Standing Magazine*.

LINDSAY GIBSON is a motivational speaker, writer, yoga instructor and spiritual joy restoration/health coach, helping to bring light back into people to promote inner healing. She is the creator of her seven-week therapeutic writing series, *Journal Back to Joy* and author of the memoir *Just Be: How my Stillborn Son Taught Me to Surrender*. Lindsay spends most of her time taking care of her two young blondie daughters and all else that motherhood entails. She is also mother to her angel son above, whose love shines through her every day. Her greatest passion is writing to inspire through heart and through Spirit.

MARIE EMMEL-FRAZER is a dedicated wife and mother of two beautiful and talented daughters and an angelic son that resides in heaven. She is happiest when in the kitchen experimenting, and can be found at www.facebook.com/winedivasonoma. Marie enjoys creating healthy, delicious meals as well as spending quality time laughing and making memories with family and friends. She is passionate about serving her community, is involved with many organizations, and has been a public speaker/spokesperson throughout the years. She lives in northern California.

NICHOLE DAVIS lives in a small town in north Georgia where she is a wife, certified surgical technologist, and mother to her son, Colson, and identical twin daughters, Callie and Coley. After Coley was born still in November of 2014, she started volunteering with two organizations; Footprints on the Heart and Remembering Our Babies, both of which she currently serves with as a board member. Her passion is to help break the silence regarding pregnancy and infant loss and to bring awareness to her community, while keeping Coley's memory alive.

PATRICIA WINKELMAN is a wife and mother of two beautiful daughters. She volunteers with various non-profits. One orgranization which is very near and dear to her heart is Compassionate Friends, a support group for bereaved parents. She resides on Olympic Peninsula in Washington with her husband and daughter.

RACHEL TENPENNY CRAWFORD is the co-founder and Chief Visionary Officer of Teamotions (www.teamotionstea.com), an emotional wellness company based in Ojai, CA. Through tea tastings, public speaking events, podcasts, and writing, Rachel teaches how to use the Teamotions line of hand-blended teas as a tool to cultivate a heart-centered approach to emotional health and well-being. As a Certified Grief Recovery Specialist®, Rachel is a passionate advocate for holistic grief recovery, emotional healing, and well-being.

RACHEL MCGRATH is an Australian who has been living in the UK for the past 10 years. There, she met and married her husband, and recently gave birth to her first child. She has authored three memoirs documenting her fertility struggles, as well as several children's fiction stories. Her first book, *Finding the Rainbow*, has won several awards in its genre. Rachel blogs at findingtherainbow.net to support women through their fertility journey.

ROSIE O'BRIEN is a teacher, wife, and loving mama to two beautiful baby girls, Ariana and Bayah, and a chocolate Labrador named Buster. She sees the importance of breaking the silence and speaks openly about losing her firstborn to stillbirth. She is happiest spending time with family and close friends. She enjoys camping, hiking, reading, and traveling. Rosie lives in northern California with her husband, Steve, daughter Bayah, and puppy, Buster.

SHARON COX is a dreamer, freedom fighter and an adventure seeker. She is a strong believer in the power of love. Growing up in South Africa taught her to recognize beauty in diversity and the importance of honoring our individual stories. She loves collecting old cameras, creating art and surrounding herself with people who live deeply. Sharon works as a chaplain and infant loss specialist in northern California.

STACEY PORTER is the founder of The Tangerine Owl Project (www.tangerineowl.org), an Illinois non-profit that offers peer support to families who have suffered infant loss in memory of her angel Delilah. Stacey devotes a majority of her time to projects and organizations that focus on advocating for maternal mental health. She is based in the north suburbs of Chicago, IL with her husband and two surviving children.

STEPHANIE TOWER is mother to three boys; sunshine child Milo, angel Oliver who died at 10 weeks of SIDS, and rainbow baby Brodie. She is a full-time mama, CPS social worker and wife to her husband Chris in Sonoma County, CA, where she was born and raised. Stephanie enjoys camping and hiking with her family, cooking, and hosting gatherings for friends and family.

TONI BRABEC is a Canadian-born, full-time working mom and wife, residing in northern California with her husband and rainbow baby boy. After the death of her first child, followed by an early miscarriage, Toni, together with her husband, is exploring ways to bring comfort and support to parents and families whose babies has been given a life-limiting or fatal diagnosis during pregnancy. Toni enjoys a good book or movie and, most of all, loves making special memories with her family like taking mini road trips or going on adventures to the park.

TRINA MCCARTNEY is a wife and the mother of four beautiful children. She is a contributor to the bereavement section of *The Compass*, a pediatric neurosurgery publication for the Stollery Children's Hospital in Edmonton, Canada. Trina is happiest making memories with her family, traveling, camping, practicing yoga, and visiting with good friends, near and far. Trina lives in Edmonton, Canada with her husband and their three children.

About the Author

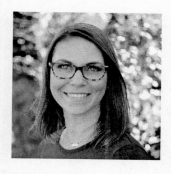

AMIE LANDS is the author of *Navigating the Unknown: An Immediate Guide When Experiencing the Loss of Your Baby* and an ongoing contributor at *Still Standing Magazine*. She is the proud founder of The Ruthie Lou Foundation as well as a Certified Grief Recovery Specialist®. Since her daughter's brief life, Amie's passion is offering hope and providing support to bereaved families. Amie lives in northern California, United States with her husband and their two sons.

www.amielandsauthor.com